Moderate Sedation for Non-Anesthesia Nurses

A Guide to Safe and Effective Sedation

M. Ron Eslinger
Captain, USN, NC, Retired
CRNA, MA, BCH

Updated May 2022

Published by Healthy Visions
M. Ron Eslinger Company
351 Market Street, Clinton, TN 37716
Phone 865-269-4616

Copyright 2019 – 2022 M. Ron Eslinger

For more information visit:
www.sedationcertification.com
www.aamsn.org

Printed in the United States of America

About the Author

Michael R. "Ron" Eslinger, RN, CRNA, MA, APN, FNGH, Captain, USN, NC, Retired, serves as Owner/CEO of Healthy Visions, a training company, and President of the American Association of Moderate Sedation Nurses, Inc. (AAMSN).

In the early 1990s, Eslinger served as a staff CRNA at Naval Hospital Jacksonville, FL. He was assigned as a committee member to establish I.V. conscious sedation policies to meet the Joint Commission Association for Healthcare Organization's standards for conscious sedation. The policies, training requirements, and competencies developed through the committee became the foundation for other navy hospitals.

Eslinger retired from the Navy in December 2003 and continued lecturing on the legal, ethical, and controversies of non-anesthesia nurse sedation. He received requests from nurses to use the sedation training program developed for non-anesthesia nurses in giving sedation. Because of these requests, Eslinger started sedation training approved for nurse continuing education credits. Later, by request, awarded a Sedation Certification (CSRN™) which evolved into the American Association of Moderate Sedation Nurses (AAMSN). The Sedation Certification training certifies that the training meets all the standards for sedation for all accreditation organizations.

Acknowledgments

Acacia pharma for their introduction of remimazolam

American Society of Anesthesiologists (ASA)

American Association of Nurse Anesthetists (AANA)

American Association of Moderate Sedation Nurses (AAMSN)

American Association for Accreditation of Ambulatory Surgery Facilities (AAAASF)

American College of Gastroenterology (ACG)

American Gastroenterological Association (AGA)

American Society for Gastrointestinal Endoscopy (ASGE)

Association of Operating Room Nurses (AORN)

HealthyVisions.com, the parent company

Michael Kost, DNP, CRNA, CHSC, for his contributions to Moderate and Procedural sedation

MyCEcredit.com, the CE Provider

Sarah Voogd, DNP, CRNA APRN, for her contribution to the advances of capnography in moderate and procedural sedation

Society of Gastroenterology Nurses and Associates (SGNA)

Richard J. Hrezo, CRNA, for his original work on toxic language 2001

Mathew Zinder, CRNA, CH, MS, for his contribution to nurse, assisted propofol sedation

Table of Contents

Chapter One **8**
    Introduction 8
    Position Statement for RN Moderate Sedation 11
    Scope of Practice for the Registered Nurse 12
    Definition of Terms 14
    Joint Commission Policy & Preparation 16
    Goals of Sedation 21
    Sedation Continuum of Care 22

Chapter Two **23**
    Protocols and standards for safe and effective sedation 23
    Role of the Sedation Nurse 23
    Assignment of ASA Physical Status 23
    American Society of Anesthesiologists (ASA) Classification 24
    Pre-Operative Nursing Assessment 25
    Mallampati Airway Classification 31
    Four Classifications 31
    Verification of Compliance with Pre-Procedure Instructions 35
    Intra-operative Nursing Actions 37

Chapter Three **41**
    Medications for Moderate Sedation 41
    Propofol Sedation: Issues and Recommendations 58

Chapter Four **69**
    Airway Assessment 69

Chapter Five **74**
    Airway Equipment 74

Chapter Six **79**
    Monitoring Vital Signs 79
    Monitoring Airway 80

Chapter Seven **84**
    Potential Complications and Interventions During Sedation 84
    Documentation Requirements During the Recovery Phase 93

Chapter Eight **96**
    Preparation for Discharge 96
    Discharge Criteria 96
    Modified Adult Aldrete Table 98

Chapter Nine **99**
    Pediatric Age-Specific Considerations 99
    Age Related Changes in Vital Signs for Children 101
    Developmental Mechanisms of Pediatric Patient Rapport 102

Chapter Ten **108**
    Geriatric Age Specific Considerations 108

Chapter Eleven **113**
    The Power of Suggestion: The Language of Nursing 113
    Words may affect the following functions: 114
    Examples of Toxic Language: 114

References **119**

Appendix **120**
   Suggested Competency Model 120
   Non-Anesthesia Providers Administering Sedation 121
   Competency Check Off Part 1 122
   Competency Check Off Part 2 123
   Sample of Informed Consent 124
   Sample Sedation Monitoring Record 126
   Conscious Sedation Pre/Post-Procedure Summary 127
   Patients Receiving Sedation Recommendations 128
   Dilaudid® 129
   Precedex 132
   CSRN™ Scope of Practice 133
   Sample Procedural Policy for Sedation 137
Index **144**

Chapter One

Introduction

The advent of same-day surgery centers and the rise in office-based procedures requiring moderate sedation rose dramatically in the 1980s and continues at a rapid pace today. Determining what constitutes sedation and what constitutes anesthesia has created political, legal, and ethical dilemmas among anesthesia providers and physicians over the determination of the patient's ASA status, the drugs used for sedation, and critical patient safety considerations that arise across a wide variety of clinical settings. Many states and nursing organizations continue to take a passive role in the oversight of sedation activities attended by registered nurses. In contrast, some organizations such as the Association of Operating Room Nurses (AORN), Society Of Gastroenterology Nurses and Associates (SGNA), and the American Association of Moderate Sedation Nurses (AAMSN) currently offer guidelines, resources and training for nurses who have had no additional training to attend to a wider range of clinical sedation scenarios.

The Joint Commission for Health Care Organizations (Joint Commission) defines moderate sedation or conscious sedation as a minimally depressed level of consciousness induced by the administration of pharmacologic agents in which the patient retains continuous and independent ability to maintain protective reflexes, a patent airway and can be aroused by physical or verbal stimulation.

Even though the Joint Commission is referenced in this writing. Ideally, the registered nurse will be knowledgeable and familiar with their institution's accrediting organization which may include: The Joint Commission, the National Integrated Accreditation for Health Care Organizations (NIAHO) also listed as DNV Health Care - Det Norske Ventas (DNV), and the Accreditation Association for Ambulatory Health Care (AAAHC). The nurse should also be familiar with the position of the American Association of Nurse Anesthetists (AANA) and the American Society of Anesthesiologists (ASA) for patient monitoring, drug administration, and protocols for dealing with potential complications or emergency situations during and after sedation.

Moderate Sedation for Non-Anesthesia Nurses Guide is designed for nurses who are involved with managing the care of patients receiving sedative or analgesic medications while undergoing invasive diagnostic or therapeutic procedures. Medication administration, patient monitoring, discharge instruction, family teaching, and patient safety concerns are all critical care elements of patients undergoing sedation.

The Sedation Guide is designed for non-anesthesia Registered Nurses working in any surgical or procedural location where sedation is given. This includes the ER, PACU, Operating Suite, Special Procedures, Gastroenterology, Endoscopy, Radiology, Ophthalmology, Plastic Surgery, and Oral Surgery suites.

Nursing personnel are consistently involved with managing patients receiving sedative or analgesic medications during invasive diagnostic or therapeutic procedures. Medication administration, patient monitoring, discharge instruction, and family teaching are primary patient safety concerns, and all are care elements performed directly by the nurse. State boards of nursing define the scope of practice with varying degrees of specificity. It is nonetheless the sole legal responsibility of each nurse to be fully familiar with their state's board of nursing policies and guidelines, independent of the wide variety of clinical settings in which moderate sedation is administered. Such settings include diagnostic/interventional radiology/cardiology settings, dental and oral surgery centers, free-standing endoscopy centers, emergency room settings, plastic surgery centers, and other outpatient settings that may or may not be associated with or located within an acute care facility.

Sedation, moderate sedation, I.V. sedation, conscious sedation, and sedation/analgesia are interchangeable. Benzodiazepines and narcotics are the most frequently used drugs for sedation. Procedural sedation is most often associated with deep sedation using anesthesia class medications such as propofol or ketamine and involving pediatrics. However, state boards of nursing, health care institutions, medical and nursing organizations have developed their own position statements concerning the administration of anesthesia class medications. They intend to use anesthesia medications such as propofol for moderate sedation. The FDA packaging directions for anesthesia class drugs and the training required to administer them is very specific but ignored by some states and some medical associations.[1] Nurses are asked to give these drugs against the package insert.

The AAMSN lists the registered nurse's responsibilities in sedation related procedures to include: being aware of their state board of nursing and their facility position statement regarding RNs giving sedation, understanding the goals of moderate sedation, differentiating between moderate and deep sedation, being knowledgeable about the medications used, knowing the side effects and unexpected outcomes, as well as performing an ongoing assessment of the patient, recognizing arrhythmias, using and interpreting pulse oximetry, and being able to intervene appropriately when oxygenation levels drop. The sedation nurse must also ensure the appropriate monitoring equipment is available and functioning correctly and verify the patient has signed the informed consent before sedation. A responsible adult will accompany the patient upon discharge. It is also the responsibility of the nurse to participate in performance improvement activities.

This guide will provide the necessary information to administer approved drugs for sedation. This guide includes proposed policies for your facility, standards of care, pharmacology, and complications related to the administration of medications, airway management, and age-specific patient assessment considerations.

This guide takes the position that registered nurses, trained and experienced in critical care and working in emergency and/or peri-anesthesia specialty areas, may be given the responsibility of administration and maintenance of moderate or conscious sedation in the presence, and by the order, of a physician. The registered nurse has the knowledge and experience to assess, interpret and intervene in the event of complications.

Position Statement for RN Moderate Sedation

Regarding the Role of the RN involved in the Management of Patients Receiving Sedation for Short-Term Therapeutic, Diagnostic or Surgical Procedures.

Even though this guide targets RNs, the same responsibilities hold true for all licensed healthcare professionals involved in sedation management.

Definition: Sedation provides a reduced level of consciousness in which the patient retains the ability to independently and continuously maintain an airway and respond appropriately to physical stimulation or verbal command.

Position: This writing teaches that registered nurses trained and experienced in critical care, emergency and/or peri-anesthesia specialty areas may be given the responsibility of administration and maintenance of sedation in the presence and by the order of a physician. The registered nurse has the knowledge and experience with medications used and the skills to assess, interpret and intervene in the event of complications. The registered nurse is an asset to the physician and enhances the quality of care provided to the patient.

When the RN has the task of monitoring the patient who is receiving sedation, a second nurse or associate should assist the physician with other complicated procedures (made so either by the severity of the patient's illness and/or the complex technical requirements of advanced diagnostic and therapeutic procedures). This is due to the importance of having the RN focus on the patient.

The registered nurse will be knowledgeable and familiar with their own institution's guidelines as well as those of the accreditation organizations for their institution. These may include the American Association of Nurse Anesthetists (AANA), the American Association of Moderate Sedation Nurses (AAMSN), and the American Society of Anesthesiologists (ASA), all of which deal with patient monitoring, drug administration, and protocols for dealing with potential complications or emergencies during and after sedation.

Scope of Practice for the Registered Nurse

It is within the scope of practice of a registered nurse to manage the care of patients receiving moderate sedation during therapeutic, diagnostic, or surgical procedures, provided the following criteria are met:

1. Administration of moderate sedation medications by non-anesthetist RNs is allowed by state laws and institutional policy, procedures, and protocol.

2. A qualified anesthesia provider or attending physician selects and orders the medications to achieve moderate sedation.

3. Guidelines for patient monitoring, drug administration, and protocols for dealing with potential complications or emergency situations are available and have been developed in accordance with accepted standards of anesthesia practice.

4. The registered nurse managing the care of the patient receiving moderate sedation shall have no other responsibilities that would leave the patient unattended or compromise continuous monitoring.

5. The registered nurse managing the care of patients receiving moderate sedation can demonstrate:

   a. Acquired knowledge of anatomy, physiology, pharmacology, and recognition of cardiac arrhythmia and complications related to moderate sedation and medications.

   b. The ability to assess total patient care requirements during moderate sedation and recovery. Physiologic measurements should include, but not be limited to, respiratory rate, oxygen saturation, blood pressure, cardiac rate and rhythm, and the patient's level of consciousness.

   c. An understanding of the principles of oxygen delivery, respiratory physiology, transport, and uptake, and demonstrate the ability to use oxygen delivery devices.

d. The ability to anticipate and recognize potential complications of moderate sedation in relation to the type of medication administered.

   e. The requisite knowledge and skills to assess, diagnose and intervene in the event of complications or undesired outcomes and to institute nursing interventions in compliance with orders (including standing orders) or institutional protocols or guidelines.

   f. Skill in airway management resuscitation.

   g. Knowledge of the legal ramifications of administering moderate sedation and/or monitoring patients receiving moderate sedation, including the RN's responsibility and liability in the event of an untoward reaction or life-threatening complication.

6. The institution or practice setting has an educational competency validation mechanism that includes evaluating and documenting the individual's knowledge, skills, and abilities related to the management of patients receiving moderate sedation. Evaluation and documentation of competency occur periodically according to institutional policy.

Definition of Terms

Minimal Sedation (Anxiolysis)

A drug-induced state during which patients respond normally to verbal commands. Although cognitive function and coordination may be impaired, ventilatory and cardiovascular functions are unaffected.

The following signs can be used to identify minimal sedation (anxiolysis):
- A normal response to verbal stimulation
- Airway unaffected
- Spontaneous ventilation unaffected
- Cardiovascular function unaffected

Moderate Sedation/Analgesia

Moderate sedation is a drug-induced depression of consciousness during which patients respond purposefully to verbal commands, either alone or accompanied by light tactile stimulation. No interventions are required to maintain a patent airway and spontaneous ventilation is adequate. Cardiovascular function is usually maintained.

The following are characteristics of moderate sedation:
- Purposeful response to verbal or tactile stimulation
- No airway intervention required
- Spontaneous ventilation adequate
- Cardiovascular function is usually maintained

Note:
Reflex withdrawal from a painful stimulus is NOT considered a purposeful response. Practitioners involved with moderate sedation must be prepared to "rescue" from deep sedation.

Deep Sedation/Analgesia

Deep sedation is a drug-induced depression of consciousness during which patients are not easily aroused but respond purposefully following repeated or painful stimulation. The ability to independently maintain ventilatory function may be impaired. Patients may require assistance in maintaining a patent airway, and spontaneous ventilation may be inadequate. Cardiovascular function is usually maintained.

The following are characteristics of deep sedation/analgesia:
- A purposeful response following repeated or painful stimulation
- Airway intervention may be required
- Spontaneous ventilation may be inadequate
- Cardiovascular function is usually maintained

Note:
Reflex withdrawal from a painful stimulus is NOT considered a purposeful response. Providers of deep sedation/analgesia must be prepared to "rescue" from general anesthesia.

Deep sedation will be performed in appropriate settings *only* by providers credentialed to provide general anesthesia.

General Anesthesia

General anesthesia is the induction of a state of unconsciousness with the absence of pain sensation over the entire body through the administration of anesthetic drugs. It is used during certain medical and surgical procedures and may include.

The ability to independently maintain ventilatory function is often impaired. Patients often require assistance in maintaining a patent airway, and positive pressure ventilation may be required because of depressed spontaneous ventilation or drug-induced depression of neuromuscular function. Cardiovascular function may be impaired. General anesthesia will be performed by credentialed anesthesia providers under the standards of anesthesia care.

Level of Sedation/Analgesia/Anesthesia

Description	Minimal Sedation	Moderate Sedation/ Analgesia	Deep Sedation/ Analgesia	General Anesthesia
Responsiveness	Normal response to verbal stimulation	Purposeful response to verbal or tactile stimulation	Purposeful response following repeated or painful stimulation	Unarousable even with painful stimulus
Airway	Unaffected	No intervention required	Intervention may be required	Intervention often required
Spontaneous Ventilation	Unaffected	Adequate	May be inadequate	Frequently inadequate
Cardiovascular Function	Unaffected	Usually maintained	Usually maintained	May be impaired

Accreditation for Health Care Organizations

- Joint Commission for Health Care Organizations
- National Integrated Accreditation for Healthcare Organizations (NIAHO) in affiliation with Det Norske Veritas (DNV)
- Health Care Accreditation Association for Ambulatory Health Care (AAAHC)
- Healthcare Facility Accreditation Program (HFAP)

Joint Commission Policy & Preparation

The Joint Commission Anesthesia/Sedation healthcare standards further require that individuals who are approved to administer any type of sedation can perform airway and cardiac rescue. It is well recognized that registered nurses trained and experienced in critical care, emergency and/or peri-anesthesia specialty areas may be given the responsibility of administration and maintenance of sedation in the presence and by the order of a physician who is present during the procedure. Although the ultimate responsibility for the patient's care lies with the procedural physician, the registered nurse must have the knowledge, skills, and experience to assess, interpret and intervene in the event of a range of complications. Even though such nurses are Advanced Cardiac Life Support (ACLS) certified and trained to resuscitate, they are not legally recognized to administer or monitor patients under general anesthesia.

Among the legal issues confronting nurses is the lack of a detailed sedation policy by some state boards of nursing. Currently, some states do not have a sedation policy for non-anesthesia nurses. Therefore, no guidelines exist for moderate sedation in those states other than what the facilities or practices themselves develop. Of equal concern is the administration of sedation to geriatric and pediatric age-specific populations with varying comorbidities or risk factors.

ACLS certification is not a Joint Commission requirement but is used as an example for institutions to use as a certification requirement.[7] Therefore, in a state which does not require ACLS certification, it is possible for a patient to receive sedation from a nurse who is not ACLS certified. For example, the American Association of Moderate Sedation Nurses (AAMSN) was contacted recently by a new nurse hire concerned that the only orientation to sedation she received was a four-page printout with no guidance or policy regarding sedation other than drug dosages and sedation definitions. Current Basic Life Support (BLS) certification was the only recommendation.

Joint Commission Guidelines

Joint Commission 2000 by Dean Smith, MD

"Qualified individuals" conducting sedations must possess education, training, and experience in:

1. **Evaluating** patients prior to moderate or deep sedation.
2. **Rescuing** patients who slip into a "deeper than desired" level of sedation or anesthesia.
3. **Managing** a compromised airway during a procedure.
4. **Handling** a compromised cardiovascular system during a procedure.

Care of Patients

TX 2   Moderate or deep sedation and ANESTHESIA are provided by qualified individuals.

TX 2.1   A presedation or ANESTHESIA assessment is preferred for each patient before beginning moderate or deep sedation and before ANESTHESIA induction.

TX 2.1.1   Each patient's moderate or deep sedation and ANESTHESIA care is planned.

TX 2.2   Sedation and ANESTHESIA options and risks are discussed with the patient and family prior to administration.

TX 2.3   Each patient's physiological status is monitored during sedation or ANESTHESIA administration.

TX 2.4   The patient's post procedure status is assessed on admission to and before discharge from the postsedation or POSTANESTHESIA recovery area.

TX 2.4.1   Patients are discharged from the postsedation or POSTANESTHESIA recovery area and the organization by a qualified licensed independent practitioner or according to criteria approved by the medical staff.

Joint Commission Standard Question

Q. Does the person administering sedation have to be qualified to monitor the patient if other staff who are present are qualified?

A. Standard PC.13.20 requires a sufficient number of staff, in addition to the person performing the procedure, be present to perform the procedure, monitor and recover the patient.

Joint Commission Policy

- *The person administering the medication must be qualified to manage the patient at whatever level of sedation or anesthesia is achieved, either intentionally or unintentionally.*
- Must be able to manage one level deeper.
- There may be a need for additional monitoring personnel, but the person administering the sedation must be qualified to monitor the patient.

Joint Commission Question – Permission to Administer Moderate Sedation

Q: Are specific privileges to administer moderate sedation required?

A: The anesthesia care standards require that the individuals who are "permitted" to administer sedation are able to perform airway & cardiac rescue.

Joint Commission Policy – Permission to Administer Moderate Sedation

Each organization is free to define how it will determine that the individuals are able to perform the required types of rescue.

Acceptable examples include, but are not limited to, ACLS certification, a satisfactory score on a written examination developed in concert with the department of anesthesiology, and a mock rescue exercise evaluated by an anesthesiologist.

The following proposed revision by the Joint Commission could affect the above recommendation that the department of anesthesiology be involved in the development of a RN certification program. The reason appears to be because many facilities doing sedation do not have Anesthesia LIPs on staff.

The Joint Commission is proposing a revision of the Anesthesia Standard. There are two proposed changes. One is to remove the requirement that a licensed independent practitioner (LIP) be involved AT ALL during the performance of surgery and sedation or anesthesia [PC.13.20]. The other change is to remove the requirement for involvement of a LIP in the planning of sedation or anesthesia [EP.11].

Joint Commission Policy – Permission to Administer Moderate Sedation

Regarding non-Licensed Independent Providers (LIPs), such as nurses, who are permitted to administer the sedation, the permission could be found in the individual's job description, or other documentation in their personnel file.

Joint Commission Policy - Perform a Time-out

The procedure is not started until all questions or concerns are resolved.

- Conduct a time-out immediately before starting the invasive procedure or making the incision.
- A designated member of the team starts the time-out.
- The time-out is standardized.
- The time-out involves the immediate members of the procedure team: the individual performing the procedure, anesthesia providers, circulating nurse, operating room technician, and other active participants who will be participating in the procedure from the beginning.
- All relevant members of the procedure team actively communicate during the time-out.
- During the time-out, the team members agree, at a minimum, on the following:
    - Correct patient identity
    - Correct site
    - Procedure to be done

- When the same patient has two or more procedures: If the person performing the procedure changes, another time-out needs to be performed before starting each procedure.

- Document the completion of the time-out. The organization determines the amount and type of documentation.

Goals of Sedation

Maintenance of adequate ventilation, homeostasis, and circulation
- A – B – C's
- An intravenous line is essential (except in some special cases of oral sedation)
- Supplemental oxygen is appropriate for most cases

Maintenance of appropriate level of consciousness
- Alteration of mood
- Still able to cooperate
- Some degree of amnesia is desirable

Promotion of comfort
- Elevation of pain threshold to produce satisfactory analgesia
- Increase patient cooperation

Ensuring patient safety by realizing the potential for *possible* consequences of:
- Respiratory depression
- Airway obstruction
- Apnea
- Hypoxia
- Hypercapnia
- Bradycardia
- Asystole
- Brain injury/brain death

Sedation Continuum of Care

Consciousness .... minimal sedation .... moderate sedation .... deep sedation .... anesthesia .... coma

The goal of the nurse and provider managing the sedation patient on this continuum is "moderate sedation."

The person monitoring the sedation must be able to rescue at any level of sedation.

Sedation Continuum of Care

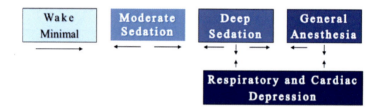

Over Sedation, "toxicity"—A definite risk; when sedation becomes deep-sedation or general anesthesia and results in respiratory and cardiac depression and if not properly treated death.

Chapter Two

Protocols and standards for safe and effective sedation

1. Motivated team
   - Patient:
     - Psychologically suitable.
     - No medical contraindications (i.e., must meet ASA Classification requirements).
     - Prepared with appropriate education.
   - Skilled providers for sedation:
     - Credentialed and privileged provider.
     - A registered nurse who has completed a competency program.
2. Appropriate time estimate of procedure:
   - Sedation is most effective for procedures requiring less than two hours to complete.
   - An alternative pain management option should be considered if the procedure is predicted to be greater than 2 hours.

Role of the Sedation Nurse

1. Pre-operative assessment
2. Intra-operative actions as defined by the procedure
3. Post-operative monitoring
4. Patient-specific discharge instructions

Assignment of ASA Physical Status

Sedation outside the main operating room is intended for either healthy patients or those with minimal illness. Before undergoing sedation, all patients are assessed by the physician and nurse performing the procedure using the American Society of Anesthesiologists (ASA) Physical Status Classification System. This system helps qualify relative risk to patients requiring sedative medications. The higher the level of classification, the more the health care team must be alert for possible sedation complications.

Adult patients classified as ASA 3 *unstable* or greater require sedation to be evaluated or delivered by an anesthesia provider.

Pediatric patients <9 months or pediatric patients classified ASA 3 *stable* or greater require sedation to be delivered by anesthesia providers.

American Society of Anesthesiologists (ASA) Classification

Class I   A normally healthy patient, i.e., no chronic illness, no regular medications.

Class II   A patient with mild systemic disease, e.g. controlled hypertension and type 2 diabetes; history of tobacco use; obesity; non-metastatic carcinoma. A well-controlled asthma patient with no recent exacerbations. A child with underlying cerebral palsy. A child with a well-controlled seizure disorder.

Class III A patient with severe systemic disease, e.g. poorly controlled hypertension; multiple medications for cardiac, respiratory and/or metabolic disorders; metastatic disease with some interference with function.

    Class III may be divided into STABLE and UNSTABLE categories. Examples are:

    Stable   Controlled insulin-dependent diabetic with hypertension and mild renal disease; a child with congenital heart disease stable on digoxin and Lasix.

    Unstable   Frequent asthma attacks needing ER visits or intubation; brittle, or difficult to control, insulin-dependent diabetic; severe COPD, on multiple inhalers and difficulty breathing in supine position.

Class IV A patient with severe systemic disease that is a constant threat to life, e.g., a metastatic disease with severe organ dysfunction; severe hypertension with angina; recent MI with continuing symptoms.

Class V A moribund patient who is not expected to survive, e.g. poorly responsive cardiogenic shock; ruptured abdominal aortic aneurysm with severe hypotension; head trauma with increasing ICP.

Class VI A declared brain-dead patient whose organs are being removed for donor purposes.

Pre-Operative Nursing Assessment

AAMSN Recommended Practice
"Each patient who will receive intravenous sedation/analgesia should be assessed physiologically and psychologically before the procedure." The assessment should be documented in the patient's medical record.

Joint Commission Standard PE.1.8.1
Any patient for whom moderate or deep sedation or anesthesia is contemplated must receive a pre-sedation or pre-anesthesia assessment.

Step 1 - Chart Review

1. Past Medical Illnesses
   - Previous medical and surgical illness.
   - Allergies.

2. Prior Surgical Procedures
   - Look at anesthesia and sedation records for information about airway management, drug reactions, and intra-anesthetic complications.
   - A previous uncomplicated procedure cannot be taken as a guarantee of a problem-free course.

3. Laboratory Studies – defined by institutional policy
   - Each patient's lab studies should be appropriate for physical status.

- Potentially fertile females between the ages of 8 and 55 <u>need</u> a urine HCG before sedation.

4. Current Medications
   - Prescription.
   - Over the counter (aspirin/ibuprofen).
   - Compliance with medication regimen.

5. Ancillary Studies (recommended)
   - 12-lead ECG for females over age 50 and for males over age 40.
   - Any patient who reports questionable information regarding the cardiac system, e.g., chest pain, SOB, high blood pressure, edema or murmur, need of an ECG is determined by the provider performing the procedure.

Step 2 - Patient Interview

1. Location, timing, privacy, and good rapport between nurse and patient are essential. Lessening stress may even decrease the amount of medication required.

2. General Health Data:

   a. Age – Identify any age-specific needs.

   b. Height and Weight (in kg).

   c. Vital Signs.

   d. Medications – Review patient's current medications and dosages, including over-the-counter ones. Ask the patient the date and time they took their last medications. Medications that should be taken with a sip of water before procedures include (e.g., anti-hypertensives, cardiac meds, antidepressants, inhalers, and bronchodilators).

e. Allergies – note actual allergic response and differentiate from an adverse reaction to the medication. Symptoms of allergic response include: urticaria, hypotension, airway edema, hives, wheezing, bronchospasm, circulatory collapse. Examples of adverse reactions are nausea, vomiting, and drowsiness.

f. Cigarette smoking – number of packs smoked per day and number of years of smoking. Cigarette smoke increases airway irritability decreases mucociliary transport and increases secretions. Smokers have higher levels of carbon monoxide in their systems, putting them at greater risk for hypoxemia.

g. Alcohol use – assess how much alcohol consumed on a daily or weekly basis. Patients with heavy/daily use may require additional sedative and analgesic medications, unless the patient has hepatic and multisystem disease associated with chronic alcohol use, in which case less medication should be used. Recovery may take significantly longer for these patients. Assess patient on the day of the procedure for signs of acute intoxication.

h. Other substance use/abuse – Assess for use of illicit substances such as cocaine or marijuana. Ask if patient taking over-the-counter stimulant or weight reduction medications, or if they are using narcotics and benzodiazepines on a regular basis. These patients may have a greater tolerance to the sedation medications that you administer.

i. Psychosocial – Assess the patient's verbal and nonverbal behaviors to establish the degree of anxiety about the procedure, ability to understand instructions and communicate verbally. Identify availability of social support systems and potential cultural barriers.

j. NPO status: Anesthesiology

Ingested Material	Minimum Fasting Period	Ingested Material	Minimum Fasting Period
Clear liquids	2h	Nonhuman milk	6h
Breast milk	4h	Light meal	6h
Infant formula	6h	Full meal / Fat	Up to 8h

k. Check on vested responsible adult escort. The adult should be present when home care instructions are reviewed with patient.

l. Menstrual history – urine HCG for potentially fertile women (check institution policy).

m. Past face, neck, oropharyngeal trauma or surgeries – Temporomandibular joint (TMJ) examination. The patient should have good TMJ mobility in case an airway needs to be inserted orally due to respiratory distress. In the adult, the distance between the upper and lower central incisors is usually 4-6 cm. Reduced TMJ mobility may be indicated by a clicking sound, pain associated with opening of the mouth, or a distance less than 4 cm upon opening. This may reveal that patient is at risk for difficult intubation due to anatomical limitations.

n. Dentition – Assess patient to identify loose, chipped, cracked or capped teeth, dental anomalies, crowns, bridges, and dentures. Knowledge of any removable items in the mouth is required in case of intubation. Be certain to document any pre-existing tooth damage to preclude later blame.

Step 3 ... Physical Exam and Review of Systems

1. Cardiovascular System

    a. History of an MI – Interval since performed. Elective procedures may be postponed until at least 6 months post-MI to decrease the incidence of reinfarction.

    b. Hypertension – Identify method of management and degree of compliance.

    c. Coronary Artery Disease – Assess for angina – if positive, have patient identify frequency, location, duration, radiation, methods of relief and whether their pattern of angina is stable.

    d. Recent cardiac surgery.

    e. Congestive heart failure – Shortness of breath at rest, with exercise or activity? Paroxysmal nocturnal dyspnea: will patient be able to lie flat for the procedure?

    f. Valvular heart disease – Auscultate for presence of murmur. Will patient require subacute bacterial endocarditis (SBE) prophylaxis before and after procedure?

    g. Cardiac dysrhythmias – Type? How does the patient tolerate it?

    h. Pacemaker or Automatic Internal Defibrillator – Underlying rhythm? Is patient pacer dependent?

    i. Cardiovascular physical assessment should include skin color, peripheral pulses, presence of edema or jugular vein distention (JVD), baseline heart rate, blood pressure and auscultation of heart sounds.

2. Pulmonary System

    a. Most sedative and analgesic medications interfere with spontaneous ventilation. Prevention of pulmonary complications requires thorough pre-procedure assessment and planning.

b. Sedation is riskier for patients with the following pulmonary conditions: Chronic Obstructive Pulmonary Disease (COPD), emphysema, bronchitis, asthma, tuberculosis, pneumonia, lung surgery, sleep apnea syndrome.

c. Assess if patient is currently having any of the following symptoms: cough, sputum production, rhinitis, sore throat, dyspnea, hemoptysis, wheezing. Notify the physician. Acute illness: Teach patient to notify clinic/physician if any of the above symptoms develop at any time prior to the procedure.

d. Extra precautions should be taken with asthmatic or chronic bronchitis patients. If the patient uses a metered-dose inhaler, they should bring it with them on procedure day. Presence of wheezing even with bronchodilator and steroid therapy should be referred to the anesthesia department or considered for rescheduling.

e. Use of O_2 at home?

f. Identify physical characteristics which may indicate the potential for difficult airway management: significant obesity, short thick neck, limited neck ROM, deviated trachea, hypognathic (recessed) jaw, hypergnathic (protruding) jaw, small mouth opening (< 3 cm), high arched palate, macroglossia (large tongue), protruding teeth, loose teeth or dentures, non-visible uvula, tonsillar hypertrophy.

Mallampati Airway Classification

Mallampati Airway Classification System – Classify the patient's airway using this system. This system is used to predict patients who may be prone to difficult intubation. The same patients are also prone to difficult airway maintenance while sedated!

- Extremely easy-to-perform, no cost, preoperative exam.
- Considered accurate predictors of subtle anatomic causes of intubation difficulty.
- Patient should sit upright with the head in a neutral position and asked to open mouth as wide as possible and to protrude the tongue as far as possible (Do not ask the patient to say "ah"). Classification can then be made as follows per visualization of the following structures in the oral cavity; uvula, facial pillars, and soft palate. A difficult endotracheal intubation is predicted for Class III & IV patients. Class III and IV require anesthesia consultation.

Four Classifications

Class I:	Soft palate, uvula, anterior and posterior tonsillar pillars.
Class II:	Soft palate, fauces, uvula.
Class III:	Soft palate, base of uvula.
Class IV:	Soft palate not visible at all.

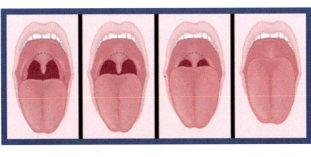

Class I   Class II   Class III   Class IV

3. Endocrine System

   a. Assess for the presence of:
      1) Diabetes – Identify type of DM and how patient manages their disease, e.g. insulin, oral agents, diet. For diabetic patients:
         - Provide clear instructions regarding their p.o. medications or insulin prior to scheduled procedure.
         - Assess patient's actual management of medications prior to procedure.
      - Make every attempt to schedule the diabetic patient as first case of the day. If they are scheduled for procedures in the afternoon, consult with anesthesia staff regarding medication regime recommendations.

      - *For patients well controlled on oral hypoglycemics who are receiving sedation for a short-term procedure (<1 hour), generally, the following instructions may be utilized:*

         - Do not take normally scheduled AM dose of oral hypoglycemic secondary to the long-term effects of possibly greater than 36 hours.
         - The morning of the procedure, a finger stick glucose is required to assess the patient's glucose level.
         - A follow-up finger stick after the procedure should be done to assess the need for intervention.

      2) *For longer procedures >1 hour and for well controlled insulin-dependent patients, the following guidelines are provided:*

         - Consultation with anesthesia staff for medication recommendations is required.
         - Patients usually receive their normal dose of NPH the evening prior to the procedure and

half their prescribed AM dose on the morning of the procedure.
- Finger stick glucose should be obtained every 30 minutes during the procedure and every hour during recovery.

DANGER: Under deep sedation signs of hypoglycemia are masked, and blood sugar may fall dangerously low.

b. Hyperthyroidism or hypothyroidism – The pharmacologic effects of sedative and analgesics may be altered in these conditions and airway management may be more difficult in both situations. The thyroid gland may be enlarged in hyperthyroidism. The tongue may be enlarged in hypothyroidism.

4. Neurologic System
Ask patient if they have a history of the following: TIA, CVA, seizure disorder or head trauma, convulsive disorders or epilepsy. Assess the following – general affect & behavior, speech pattern alterations, level of consciousness, orientation and gait. If local anesthesia is to be used, it is important to determine the presence of pre-existing numbness or weakness.

5. Hepatic System
Assess patient for medical history of hepatitis or cirrhosis. Patients with impaired liver function may exhibit altered drug metabolism and elimination, which can result in either resistance to sedation medications or increased sensitivity to the medications.

6. Gastrointestinal System
Assess the patient for the following symptoms and conditions: nausea, vomiting, diarrhea, constipation, GI bleeding, GI surgery or Gastric reflux. A histamine blocker may be ordered for the patient with gastric reflux. A non-particulate antacid, such as Bicitra, may also be considered.

7. Renal System
    Renal disease impairs excretion of sedation medications and their metabolites. Assess the patient for renal insufficiency or renal failure. These patients will probably require pre-procedure consultation and may not be candidates for nurse-monitored sedation. The nurse will need to collaborate with the physician to closely regulate the patient's fluid status. If the patient has an AV fistula (peripheral vascular cannulation site), avoid blood pressure measurements and IV insertions on that extremity.

    Assess the patient's fluid status as indicated by the length of NPO status, urine output, skin turgor, mucous membrane appearances, blood pressure, and heart rate.

8. Musculoskeletal System
    Ask the patient if they have a history of arthritis or recent fractures. Assess level of mobility, range of motion, muscle strength and neurovascular status in affected areas.

9. Integumentary System - comprises the skin and its appendages (including hair and nails). Assess skin color, temperature, turgor, and integrity.

10. Anesthesia and Surgical History
    Ask the patient what surgeries or procedures they have had in the past and type of anesthesia.

    Ask whether the patient had any complications associated with past anesthesia including reactions to medications, nausea and vomiting, or airway difficulties. *Any patient reporting a history of airway difficulties should be referred to anesthesia staff for their recommendations.*

11. Review of Laboratory Data
    Review results of pre-laboratory data as ordered by the physician. Verify that a pregnancy test according to institution policy has been completed on all females of childbearing age. Notify the physician of any abnormalities.

Sedation in the pregnant patient requires obstetric and anesthesia consultation.

Verification of Compliance with Pre-Procedure Instructions

1. Informed Consent: The physician is responsible for explaining the proposed procedure, potential complications of the procedure, use of sedation, and potential risks and alternatives to sedation. *Verify that informed consent has been obtained before administration of any sedation.*

2. NPO Status: Analgesics and sedatives have an inherent side effect of nausea and vomiting.

   Additionally, patients may enter a state of deep sedation and lose protective reflexes that protect them from aspiration of gastric contents. The goal for the pre-procedure patient undergoing sedation is to prevent vomiting and aspiration of gastric contents by ensuring minimal gastric contents.

3. Procedure-specific instructions: Assess if patient completed activities specific to the procedure such as showers, enemas and medications.

4. Escort: Stress the necessity of identifying an adult non-medical attendant to escort *and stay* with patient at home post sedation. For some patients and types of procedures, it is recommended that the patient have home assistance for 12-24 hours after the procedure. Identify the presence of the patient's escort on the day of the procedure and document their presence and their name. Do not begin sedation if the escort did not accompany the patient.

5. Pre-Procedure Teaching: Teaching should include at home preparation for the procedure, NPO status, procedure specific preparation such as surgical preps, medication use, intra-procedure expectations about the procedure and the use of sedation, post-procedure expectations including immediate recovery, discharge instructions and the need for an escort.

6. However, you may not meet the patient until the day of the procedure, so assess **FIRST** what the patient already knows, and address additional learning needs. The goals of pre-op teaching are to increase patient compliance during and after the procedure and decrease the patient's anxiety.

   Patient teaching should also cover the following:

   a. Intra-procedure events
      - Length of procedure, room temperature, positioning for the procedure and safety measures.
      - Inform the patient whether they will not be able to move certain parts of their body during the procedure.
      - Infection control measures need IV access, types of monitoring equipment that will be used (e.g. pulse oximeter, cardiac monitor, and automatic BP cuff).
      - Sedation medications that will be used and the expected effects of those medications. Tell the patient the following: They will not be asleep during the procedure but should feel drowsy and relaxed; they may not remember the procedure later, and that you will be talking with them throughout the entire procedure.
      - Expected sensations during the procedure. If the procedure is expected to cause discomfort, let the patient know they will be given medication to lessen the pain (although it may not relieve it entirely). Identify a method they can use to let you know if they need more pain relief.

   b. Post-procedure (recovery) events
      - Sensations, length of time and how they will be monitored
      - Discharge criteria that must be met before discharge

The pre-procedure assessment and teaching must be documented on the appropriate form before administering sedation medications.

Intra-operative Nursing Actions

1. Continuous IV access
   A continuous infusion of IV fluids using a recommended 20G catheter or larger for adults (Check institution policy, some may be different) should be used and maintained throughout the sedation and recovery period. See facility policy.

2. Oxygen delivery
   Oxygen must be readily available for administration by mask or nasal cannula but need not be utilized if oxygen saturation remains at a satisfactory level in the judgment of the attending provider or as stated by institution policy.

3. Monitoring and documentation

   Assess:
   - Respiratory: Rate & depth of respirations, patency of airway – most respiratory problems associated with sedation are caused by the effect of medications, which decrease the rate and depth of ventilations or impair airway patency. These effects usually occur before pulse oximetry readings fall. Listen for equal, bilateral breath sounds and adequacy of tidal volume. The patient should have a minimal SpO_2 of 95% on room air or supplemental oxygen.

   - Pulse: Periodically assess heart rate, skin temperature, color, and capillary refill. Most medications used during sedation have minimal effects on the heart rate and blood pressure if the patient is in the supine position. Meperidine may cause an increase in heart rate; all other narcotics tend to decrease the heart rate.

- Blood Pressure: Use the appropriately sized cuff, assess every 5 minutes throughout the procedure; more frequently if aberrations are noted.

- Cardiac monitoring: The patient will be monitored continuously until discharge criteria are met. The monitoring RN will stay with the patient continuously during the procedure. According to the Joint Commission the RN monitoring the patient should not be engaged in tasks that would compromise continuous monitoring. Print a pre and post sedation rhythm strip and include any arrhythmia activity or events.

- Level of consciousness (LOC): It is important to assess and document baseline LOC prior to the initiation of sedation. During sedation and recovery, LOC will be documented at least every 15 minutes.

To assess:

- Ask patient to take a deep breath. This not only assesses their ability to follow a verbal command, but also causes chest expansion and helps prevent hypoventilation.

- Ask the patient a simple question that requires them to verbalize.

- The optimally sedated patient will be drowsy, close their eyes, but should be aroused easily when you call their name or gently shake them. Speech may be slightly slurred.

- Patients may momentarily react to a painful stimulus. Be aware that sedation may result in disinhibition and the patient may make purposeful movements to remove painful stimulus.

- The following signs are indicative of deepening levels of sedation: Slurred speech; becoming less responsive, more lethargic and unarousable. Should these occur, notify the physician immediately and monitor the patient for potential respiratory depression.

Documentation:
The following scale may be used to document LOC during the sedation procedure and recovery:

1. Alert, awake, oriented.
2. Occasionally drowsy, easy to arouse.
3. Frequently drowsy, able to arouse.
4. Sleeping, slow to arouse.
5. Somnolent, unable to arouse.

Other aspects to monitor include anxiety, pain and/or restlessness. Restlessness may indicate anxiety or pain; however, it might also be an early indicator of hypoxemia or a pre-syncopal episode. Hence, if your patient becomes restless, assess for multiple causes.

Requirements:
Assessment and documentation of vital signs (including Heart rate and blood pressure), respiratory rate and SpO_2 every 5 minutes during a procedure due to the potent effects of benzodiazepines and narcotics on the circulatory system. Level of consciousness will be documented at least every 15 minutes.

4. Medication administration: Administer and document medications ordered by the provider.

5. Provide nursing support interventions during procedure.

- Talk to the patient using therapeutic, positive and reassuring language. Avoid conversations in the room which ignore the patient. Avoid conversations which might be misinterpreted by a sedated patient.
- Keep the patient informed of the progress of the procedure.
- Touch the patient gently when assessing ventilations, skin temperature, LOC, or when reassuring them.
- Attend to basic comfort needs of the patient, such as repositioning.
- Observe the patient for nonverbal indicators of pain and anxiety.

6. Report these observations to the physician immediately:

- Restlessness: See above.
- Cyanosis: A late sign of hypoxemia.
- Pallor: Patients experiencing vasovagal symptoms are likely to become very pale.
- Flushing: Is a possible sign of a developing allergic reaction.
- Diaphoresis: Consider the possibility of myocardial ischemia. Assess for chest pain. Check for changes in vital signs and the ECG (look for ST segment elevation, T wave depression or inversion).
- Nausea: Check for causes including narcotics, pain, hypotension, vagal episodes, anxiety and hypoglycemia.

Be prepared to look for causative factors rather than treating the symptoms themselves. For example, if nausea is caused by hypotension, it would be entirely inappropriate to treat the patient with an anti-nausea drug such as Droperidol or Phenergan which has properties that can drop the blood pressure even further. If the patient is restless do not automatically treat for pain.

Chapter Three

Medications for Moderate Sedation

Introduction: There is no single medication that will meet all needs for sedation. In most cases, combinations of medications are administered.

Prescribing and ordering

The Joint Commission requires organizations to institute formal procedures for limiting the risk associated with prescribing and ordering medications. The standards identify ten specific areas that health care facilities are required to address; seven are relevant to anesthesia and conscious sedation.

The seven standards are:

1. Distribution, administration and/or disposal of controlled medications, such as narcotics and sedatives or hypnotics, including adequate documentation and record-keeping, as required by state and federal law.

2. Proper storage, distribution, and control of investigational medications and those in clinical trials

3. Situations in which all or some of the patient's medication orders must be permanently or temporarily concealed and mechanisms for reinstating them.

4. "As needed" (PRN) prescriptions or orders and times of dose administration.

5. Control of sample drugs.

6. Distribution of medications to patients at discharge

7. Procurement, storage, control, and distribution of prepackaged medications obtained from outside sources (CAMH, August 1997 update, TX-21)

The most frequently prescribed sedation/analgesia medications are listed here.

1. **Benzodiazepines** – Specific Agents: Diazepam (Valium), Midazolam (Versed), Remimazolam, Lorazepam (Ativan), Alprazolam (Xanax), Triazolam (Halcion)

    - These are the most widely used drugs for sedation.

    - Probably work in the limbic system and amygdala of the brain, where fear, anxiety and apprehension arise.

    - Attach to receptor sites in the cerebral cortex, enhancing gamma-aminobutyric acid (GABA) and inhibiting excitatory impulses: anxiolysis...reduction of anxiety; amnesiac...reduces ability to recall events surrounding administration; anti-convulsive...stops seizures; skeletal muscle relaxation; sedative...hypnotic in large doses.

    - Patients who chronically take Cimetidine (Tagamet) or Ranitidine (Zantac) are especially susceptible to benzodiazepine overdose. These H-2 blocking drugs may dramatically increase the sedative effect of even small doses of benzodiazepines.

    - Narcotics (when given in conjunction with benzodiazepines) are great potentiators of respiratory depression (significant synergistic effect).

    a) **Diazepam (Valium)**

Route	Onset of Action	Peak Effect	Duration of Action
IV	2-5 minutes	3-5 minutes	15-60 mins.
Oral	30 - 90 min.	60 minutes	3-8 hours

    Kost p. 103, 2020

    1. Adult dose: 0.05 – 0.15 mg/kg titrated in 1 to 2 mg increments; 1 – 2 mg IV may be titrated over 2 minutes

prior to procedure. It should be injected until the desired effect is achieved (slurred speech)—no rapid or single bolus injections—generally, 10 to 20 mg in 60 minutes; 10 mg when administered with narcotic.

2. Pediatric dose: 0.1 – 0.3 mg/kg.

3. Potential adverse reactions: phlebitis at site of injection, bradycardia, hypotension, respiratory depression and apnea, agitation, confusion, hiccups, diplopia, rash, urticaria

4. Avoid extravasation as the drug is caustic to tissue.

5. It may be diluted with normal saline only. **Do not mix with any other drug.**

6. Midazolam is generally preferable to Diazepam due to Midazolam's decreased duration and easier titratability.

7. Reversal agent: Flumazenil (Romazicon) will reverse the respiratory effects of Diazepam overdose.

b) Midazolam (Versed)

Route	Onset of Action	Peak Effect	Duration of Action
IV	1 - 2 minutes	3 – 5 minutes	10-30 min
IM	10 - 15 minutes	20-45 minutes	60-120 min
Oral	15-50 minutes	35-45 minutes	60-90 min

Kost, p. 96, 2020

1. Midazolam is a potent, short-acting drug that *must be given slowly by IV;* administration over two minutes is recommended.

2. Dilution: May dilute to the desired concentration with D5W or NS.

3. Recommend concentration of 0.25 mg/ml, with an administration rate no faster than 0.5 mg over 2 minutes.

4. Dosage recommendations for sedation:

   Adult: Initial dose of 1-2 mg IV over 2 minutes just before the beginning of the procedure. Must titrate to effect (slurred speech) by giving additional IV doses over 2 minutes. In general, do not exceed the total dose of 3.0 mg; however, you may continue to titrate higher doses if needed to obtain an effect. Wait at least 2 minutes after each medication administration to determine the effect.

   Geriatric or patients with impaired pulmonary/hepatic function: Initial dose 0.25mg-0.5mg IV over 2 minutes. The maximum total dose is 2.0 mg. Titrate to effect.

   Pediatric: 0.025 – 0.05 mg/kg IV over 2 minutes. Maximum total dose 0.1 mg /kg. Titrate to effect.

5. Contraindications: Do not give Midazolam to persons with known hypersensitivities to the drug. Do not give to patients with acute narrow-angle glaucoma and shock. Reduce dosage for patients with alcohol intoxication or a history of COPD.

6. Adverse Reactions: Respiratory depression, coughing, hypotension, bronchospasm, laryngospasm, PVCs, tachycardia, bradycardia, nausea, hiccups, vomiting, urticaria, pain at infusion site, apnea, cardiac arrest.

7. Reversal agent: Flumazenil (Romazicon) will reverse the respiratory effects of Midazolam overdose.

Sublingual midazolam for adult sedation (Use the 5 mg/ml Versed concentration):

1.0 mg is 0.2 cc	3.0 mg is 0.6 cc
1.5 mg is 0.3 cc	3.5 mg is 0.7 cc
2.0 mg is 0.4 cc	4.0 mg is 0.8 cc
2.5 mg is 0.5 cc	4.5 mg is 0.9 cc

Use the top row to calculate the dose in mgs by using the weight and age of the patient.

An 80 to 100-pound patient who is 30 to 49 years old would receive 2.5 mgs.

Weight in Pounds	Age 30-49	Age 50	Age 60	Age 70+
80-100	2.5 mgs	2.5 mgs	2.0 mgs	2.0 mgs
110 – 150	3.0 mgs	3.0 mgs	2.5 mgs	2.5 mgs
155 – 180	3.5 mgs	3.5 mgs	3.0 mgs	3.0 mgs
185 – 210	4.0 mgs	4.0 mgs	3.5 mgs	3.5 mgs
215 – 250	4.5 mgs	4.5 mgs	4.0 mgs	4.0 mgs
255+	5.0 mgs	5.0 mgs	4.5 mgs	4.5 mgs

c) Remimazolam (Byfavo®)

Route	Onset of Action	Peak Effect	Duration of Action
IV	1 – 1.5 minutes	3 – 3.5 minutes	37-53 min

Byfavo package insert

Median time to fully alert: 11.0-14.0 minutes

1. Remimazolam is a benzodiazepine indicated for the induction and maintenance of procedural sedation in adults undergoing procedures **lasting 30** minutes or less.

2. Only personnel trained in the administration of procedural sedation and not involved in the diagnostic or therapeutic procedure should administer Byfavo.

3. Only personnel trained in the administration of procedural sedation and not involved in the conduct of the diagnostic or therapeutic procedure should administer Byfavo.

4. Remimazolam (Byfavo) has been associated with hypoxia, bradycardia, and hypotension. Continuously monitor vital signs during sedation and during the recovery period.

5. Resuscitative drugs and age- and size-appropriate equipment for bag-valve-mask–assisted ventilation must be immediately available during administration of Byfavo.

6. Concomitant to benzodiazepines, including remimazolam, and opioid analgesics, may result in profound sedation, respiratory depression, coma, and death. The sedative effect of intravenous remimazolam can be accentuated by concomitantly administered CNS depressant medications, including propofol and other benzodiazepines. Continuously

monitor patients for respiratory depression and depth of sedation.

7. Dosage recommendations for sedation:

    - Adult Induction: Administer 5 mg intravenously over 1-minute

    - Maintenance (as needed) At least 2-minutes must elapse before administration of any supplemental dose and assessment of level of sedation

    - Maintenance dose is 2.5 mg intravenously over 15 seconds.

    - For ASA III and IV, Administer 2.5 my to 5 mg intravenously over 1-minute based on the patient's general condition.

    - Maintenance for ASA III and IV: Administer 1.25 mg to 2.5 mg intravenously over 15 seconds.

8. Contraindications: Do not use remimazolam in patients with a history of severe hypersensitivity reaction to dextran 40 or products containing dextran 40.

9. Adverse Reactions: Respiratory depression, coughing, hypotension, bronchospasm, laryngospasm, PVCs, tachycardia, bradycardia, nausea, hiccups, vomiting, urticaria, pain at infusion site, apnea, cardiac arrest.

10. Reversal agent: Flumazenil (Romazicon) will reverse the respiratory effects of remimazolam overdose.

11. Preparation and Administration of remimazolam (Byfavo)

    - Once removed from packaging, protect vials from light

- To reconstitute Byfavo for injection:

- Add 8.2 mL sterile 0.9% Sodium Chloride Injection, USP, to the vial; direct the stream of the solution toward the wall of the vial

- Gently swirl the vial (do not shake) until the contents are fully dissolved.

- The reconstituted product will deliver a final concentration of 2.5 mg/mL solution of Byfavo.

- After 8 hours, discard any unused portion

d) Lorazepam (Ativan)
- Uses – Anxiolysis, Sedation.
- Absorption – Gastrointestinal, prompt.
- Metabolism – Hepatic.
- Excretion – Principally in urine.
- Discussion – Anterograde and retrograde amnesia.
- Distributed in 0.5 mg, 1 mg, 2 mg tabs.
- Dose – Children > 12 years: 0.05 mg/kg; Adults 1 – 10 mg.
- Unlabeled use in children younger than 12 years.

Lorazepam (Ativan)

Route	Onset of Action	Peak Effect	Duration of Action
IV	1-5 minutes	15-20 minutes	6-24 hours
IM	15-30 minutes	15 - 60 minutes	6-24 hours
PO	1-6 hours	120 minutes	6-24 hours

Omogui, p. 106

e) **Alprazolam (Xanax)**
   - Use – Anxiolysis.
   - Dose – 0.25 – 0.5 mg.
   - Absorption – Gastrointestinal, prompt.
   - Metabolism – Hepatic.
   - Excretion (half-life) – Urine; 12 – 15 hours.
   - Distributed in 0.25, 0.5, 1.0, 2.0 mg tab; Liquid 1 mg/ml.

Route	Onset of Action	Peak Effect	Half-Life
PO	1-2 hours	120 minutes	12-15 hours
IM	15-30 minutes	15 - 60 minutes	6-24 hours
PO	1-6 hours	120 minutes	6-24 hours

Malamed, p. 108

f) **Triazolam (Halcion)**
   - Sedation is off-label use.
   - Use – Insomnia.
   - Dose – Adult 0.5 mg per oral route.
   - The relative potency is 0.1 mg.
   - Absorption – Gastrointestinal, prompt.
   - Metabolism: Hepatic.
   - Excretion (half-life): Urine; 1.5 – 5.5 hours.

Route	Onset of Action	Peak Effect	Half-Life
PO	1 hour	1.3 hours	1.5-5.5 hours

Malamed, p. 107

2. **Reversal agent for Benzodiazepines:** Flumazenil (Romazicon)

Flumazenil (Romazicon):

Route	Onset of Action	Peak Effect	Duration of Action
IV (bolus or infusion)	1 - 2 minutes	6-10 minutes (but 80% of the maximum response is seen within 3 minutes). **Call anesthesia** if there is no desired clinical response with the administration of the initial 1 mg.	45 - 90 minutes

Kost, p. 109

a. Specific benzodiazepine antagonist, used for complete or partial reversal of the sedative effects of benzodiazepines, management of benzodiazepine overdose

b. Administration Technique:

IV bolus:
- Phase One: Initially, 0.2 mg IV over 15 seconds to one minute. If the patient does not reach the desired level of consciousness after 45 seconds, proceed to Phase Two.
- Phase Two: Repeat dose at one-minute intervals until a cumulative dose of 1 mg has been administered (includes initial dose in phase one). If no response to treatment is noted, call anesthesia for assistance.

IV infusion:
30-60 ug/minute (0.5-1 ug/kg/min). Total dose not to exceed 3 mg/hour.

c. Special considerations:
- Individualized dosage is required; the manufacturer does not recommend administering Flumazenil to patients under the age of 18.
- Flumazenil-induced seizures were reported in patients with chronic physical dependence on benzodiazepines or

patients recently undergoing multiple procedures requiring large doses of benzodiazepines.
- Patients who have responded to Flumazenil should be carefully monitored (up to 120 minutes) for re-sedation.
- Administration of Flumazenil via a large vein is recommended to avoid pain and inflammation at the injection site.
- Overdose: Excessive doses result in anxiety, agitation, increased muscle tone, and possible convulsions.

d. Adverse effects:
- Respiratory – the return of respiratory depression, which has exceeded the therapeutic effects of Flumazenil.
- Cardiovascular – cutaneous vasodilation, sweating, flushing, dysrhythmias, bradycardia, tachycardia and hypertension.
- CNS – dizziness, headache, abnormal or blurred vision, confusion and convulsions.

3. **Narcotics/Opioid Agonists:** Morphine Sulfate, Meperidine, and Fentanyl

a) **Morphine Sulfate** - Binds opiate receptors in CNS, altering the perception of and emotional response to pain.

Route	Onset of Action	Peak Effect	Duration of Action
IV	5-10 minute	20 minutes	4-5 hours
IM	10-30 minutes	30-60 minutes	4-5 hours

Kost, p. 101, 2020

1. Dosage/Administration – **Adults:** 0.03 – 0.1 mg/kg in 1 mg incremental IV. Must give slowly and titrate to individual response. Assess the patient continuously for signs and symptoms of pain and give additional doses for increasing pain levels. Decrease dosage if given to elderly or debilitated patients and patients with renal or hepatic disease. Dilute with 5 ml of sterile water or NS and give

slowly. May repeat every 15 minutes. The total dosage is 10 mg in 60 minutes.

Pediatrics: 0.05 – 0.1 mg/kg IV, titrated to effect. See appendix.

2. Adverse Reactions:
   - Respiratory effects – respiratory depression, bronchospasm, laryngospasm
   - Cardiovascular effects – hypotension, hypertension, bradycardia, arrhythmias
   - CNS effects – euphoria, dysphoria, somnolence, syncope
   - GI effects – nausea, vomiting, constipation, biliary tract spasm
   - GU – urinary retention.
   - Integumentary – pruritus/local tissue irritation, urticarial, skin wheals
   - Musculoskeletal – chest wall rigidity (all narcotics can cause rigidity)

3. Reversal Agent: Naloxone (Narcan) will reverse the respiratory and cardiovascular effects of morphine sulfate overdose.

b) Meperidine Hydrochloride (Demerol) - Binds with opiate receptors in the CNS, altering perception and emotional response to pain. *Rare but still used by some institutions.*

Route	Onset of Action	Peak Effect	Duration of Action
IV	1 - 5 minutes	5-7 minutes	2-4 hours
IM	10 – 15 minutes	30-50 minutes	2-4 hours
Oral	15-45 minutes	60 - 90 minutes	2-4 hours

Kost, p. 99, 2020

1. Dosage/Administration – **Adults**: 25 mg slow IVP. Slowly titrate in 25 mg increments to individual patient response. The total dose for nursing administration is 100 mgs in 60 minutes.

    - Reduce dosage and rate of administration in patients who are elderly, debilitated, have renal or hepatic disease, or who have hypothyroidism.
    - Contraindicated in patients on Monoamine oxidase inhibitors (MAOI's). Isocarboxazid (Marplan), Phenelzine (Nardil), Selegiline (Emsam, Eldepryl, Zelapar), Tranylcypromine (Parnate)
    - Severe and even fatal reactions have been known to occur.
    - **Pediatric**: 1 – 1.5 mg/kg. Titrate dose to individual response. Max. dose 100 mgs.

2. Adverse Reactions:

    - Respiratory effects – severe respiratory depression and arrest. Use with caution in patients with COPD, asthma, corpulmonale, decreased respiratory function, hypoxia or hypercapnia.
    - Cardiovascular effects – orthostatic hypotension, bradycardia, tachycardia, palpitations, syncope, shock, cardiac arrest
    - CNS effects – euphoria, dysphoria, weakness, sedation, convulsions, agitation, tremors, uncoordinated muscle movements, transient hallucinations, disorientation and visual disturbances
    - GI – dry mouth, constipation, biliary spasm, nausea, and vomiting.
    - Integumentary – flushing, pruritus/local tissue irritation (histamine release), urticarial, skin wheals, and local irritation.
    - GU – urinary retention.

- Special considerations – this drug must be titrated to effect and administered slowly to prevent the occurrence of adverse reactions.

3. Reversal Agent: Naloxone (Narcan) will reverse the respiratory and cardiovascular effects of Meperidine overdose.

c) **Fentanyl Citrate (Sublimaze)** – Binds with opiate receptors in CNS, altering the perception of and emotional response to pain.
   - 75-100 times more potent than morphine
   - Dose 0.7-1mcg/kg
   - Titrate in 25mcg increments

Route	Onset of Action	Peak Effect	Duration of Action
IV	1-2 minutes	5-15 minutes	30-60 minutes
Trans-mucosal	5-15 minutes	20–30 minutes	1-2 hours

Kost, p. 102, 2020

1. Dosage/Administration – **Adults:** 25-100mcg slow IV injection into IV infusion line over 1-2 minutes is required. Titrate 25 mcg at a time. The total recommended dose for nursing administration is 200 mcg for a healthy young adult.
   - Reduce dosage and rate of administration in patients who are elderly, debilitated, or have renal or hepatic disease.
   - **Pediatric:** 0.5 – 2 mcg/kg. Titrate to individual response.

2. Adverse Reactions:
   - Respiratory effects – potent respiratory depression, apnea. Use caution with patients with COPD or other respiratory compromises.
   - Cardiovascular effects – hypotension, bradycardia, tachycardia, palpitations, syncope, shock, cardiac arrest.

- CNS effects – euphoria, dysphoria, weakness, sedation, agitation, tremors, seizures, and use with caution in patients with increased intracranial pressure.
- GI effects – nausea, vomiting, delayed gastric emptying, biliary tract spasm.
- Musculoskeletal – may cause muscular rigidity of the thorax to the point that ventilation (spontaneous or controlled) is impossible. A muscle relaxant can be used for treatment, but only by anesthesia providers; therefore, treat with Naloxone (Narcan).
- Special considerations – Fentanyl must be titrated to effect and administered slowly to prevent the occurrence of adverse reactions. **DO NOT** mix with barbiturates.

3. Reversal Agent: Naloxone (Narcan) will reverse the respiratory and cardiovascular effects of a fentanyl overdose. Reversal brought on too rapidly may cause nausea, sweating, and hypertension.

4. **Reversal Agent for Narcotics**

Naloxone Hydrochloride (Narcan)

Route	Onset of Action	Peak Effect	Duration of Action
IV	2 minutes	5-15 minutes	30-45 minutes

Kost, p. 108, 2020

1. Description: Naloxone is a pure opioid antagonist with no agonist activity. It reverses respiratory depression, hypotension, hypercapnia, sedation, and euphoria associated with the administration of narcotics.

2. Dosage/Administration – Naloxone injection is a sterile solution for intravenous, and intramuscular administration in three concentrations of 0.02 mg,

0.4 mg, and 1 mg of naloxone hydrochloride per ml. pH is adjusted to 3.5 ± 0.5 with hydrochloric acid.

- **Adult:** Initial dose 0.04 mg – 2 mg titrated in small increments. Dilute 0.4 mg amp of Narcan to 10cc total volume. The dose is 0.04 mg or 40 mcg per cc. Give this reversal 1cc at a time, with at least 2-3 minutes between doses. This titration will allow one to bring the patient up to a safe respiratory rate without reversing analgesia or causing severe CV problems. If no response is observed after 2 mg has been administered, the diagnosis of narcotic induced toxicity should be questioned. Total dosage for nursing administration – 2 mg.

- **Pediatric:** Initial dose 0.01 mg. If the initial dose does not result in desired clinical reversal. Administer a subsequent dose of 0.01 mg. If this does not result in the desired effect, administer 0.1 mg/kg. The total dosage for nursing administration in pediatric patients is 0.2 mg/kg.

3. Adverse Reactions:

- Respiratory effects – pulmonary edema.
- Cardiovascular effects – hypotension, hypertension, arrhythmias, ventricular tachycardia, and ventricular fibrillation
- CNS effects – excitement, tremors, seizures, reversal of analgesia.
- GI – nausea, vomiting
- Special considerations – titrate slowly to the desired effect. Complete reversal from higher doses will result in a total reversal of analgesia with other effects, including hypertension, excitation, and tachycardia. Monitor the patient closely in the post-procedure period for re-sedation. Additional doses of Naloxone may be required.

If the initial sedative/narcotic is properly titrated to effect, the reversal should not be needed. However, if it is required, usually small doses are adequate. The larger doses found in resources are indicated for significant overdoses, as seen in obtunded/comatose patients.

5. *Anesthesia Medications*

Propofol (Diprivan)
Classification: sedative-hypnotic. Propofol produces rapid hypnosis with minimal excitation.

Route	Onset of Action	Peak Effect	Duration of Action
IV	40 seconds	1 minute	5 – 10 minutes

Kost, p. 105, 2020

1. Dosage/Administration – **Adult dose**: 25 – 50mg (0.5 – 1 mg/kg) IV, administered in 10 mg increments over several minutes. Pain on injection decreases with IV lidocaine, 0.1 mg/kg, added to the propofol emulsion. A strict aseptic technique must be maintained in handling, as propofol is preservative-free and will support bacterial growth. Propofol injection should be prepared for single patient use only, just before the initiation of each procedure. Discard after open for 6 hours.

   Pediatric dose: 0.5 – 1.0 mg/kg infused slowly and titrated to the desired effect.

2. Adverse Reactions:
   - Respiratory effects – respiratory depression, apnea, hiccup, bronchospasm, laryngospasm
   - Cardiovascular effects –hypotension, arrhythmia, tachycardia, bradycardia, hypertension
   - CNS effects – headache, dizziness, euphoria, myoclonic/clonic movement, seizures, and sexual illusions.

- GI effects - nausea, vomiting, abdominal cramps

- Special considerations – propofol must be titrated to effect and administered slowly to prevent the occurrence of adverse reactions. Reduce dose in elderly, hypovolemic, and high-risk patients. Potentiation occurs when combined with narcotic analgesics and CNS depressants. There is no pharmacologic reversal agent for Propofol.

3. Propofol has anxiolytic properties, which may be related to several neuromodulator systems. Moreover, it has antioxidant, immunomodulatory, analgesic, antiemetic, and neuroprotective effects.[13]

4. When used for ventilator support, propofol injectable emulsion should not be infused for longer than five days without providing a drug holiday to replace estimated or measured urine zinc losses safely.

5. In patients at risk for renal impairment, urinalysis and urine sediment rate should be checked before initiation of sedation and then monitored on alternate days during sedation.

6. Since propofol injectable emulsion is formulated in an oil-in-water emulsion, elevations in serum triglycerides may occur when DIPRIVAN Injectable Emulsion is administered for extended periods of time. Patients at risk of hyperlipidemias should be monitored for increases in serum triglycerides or serum turbidity.

Propofol Sedation: Issues and Recommendations

Using Propofol (Diprivan) to sedate patients during endoscopic and other diagnostic procedures is gaining momentum in many hospitals, outpatient surgery centers, and physician offices. In trained hands, Propofol offers many advantages over other drugs used for sedation because it:

- It has a rapid onset (about 40 seconds) and a short duration of action
- Allows patients to wake up, recover, and return to baseline activities and diet sooner than some other sedation agents.
- Reduces the need for opioids, thus resulting in less nausea and vomiting.

Trained nurses in most critical care settings often administer propofol safely to intubated and ventilated patients. However, some practitioners have been lulled into a false sense of security, allowing the drug's good safety profile to influence their beliefs that propofol is safer than it really is. In untrained hands, propofol can be dangerous, even deadly. Administration to a nonventilated patient by a practitioner who is not trained in the use of drugs that can cause deep sedation and general anesthesia is not safe, even if the drug is given under the direct supervision of the physician performing the procedure. [2] After all, how much supervision can the physician provide if he or she is focused on the procedure itself? Not enough, as the following events show:

1. Believing that propofol was "used all the time in ICU," a gastroenterologist asked a nurse to prepare "10 mL" (10 mg/mL) of the drug for a patient undergoing endoscopy in his room. The nurse obtained the drug from an automated dispensing cabinet via override before transcribing the order to the patient's record. Another nurse who was trained in the use of moderate sedation, but not deep sedation or anesthesia, assisted the gastroenterologist. After questioning the physician about the dose (100 mg is a high dose), she began administering the Propofol via an infusion pump. The patient suddenly experienced respiratory arrest. Fortunately, ICU staff were able to help with the emergency and quickly intubated and ventilated the patient.

2. Another case involved a physician who thought he could safely administer Propofol himself while performing a breast augmentation. Unfortunately, his patient, a young woman,

died of hypoxic encephalopathy because he failed to notice the patient's rapidly declining respiratory status, as had his surgical assistant, who was not qualified to monitor patients under deep sedation or anesthesia.[3]

3. Nurses have also been asked to administer "a little more" propofol if the patient moved after the anesthesiologist left the room. In these cases, the anesthesiologist would leave the Propofol syringe and needle in the IV port after placing the block and leave the nurses in the room to monitor the patient alone. Initially, the nurses reluctantly complied. Later, they brought the issue to the attention of hospital leaders, citing that they were worried about the safety of this practice.[2]

There are several compelling reasons why all healthcare providers should be worried about nurse-administered propofol.

Strict Product Labeling:
AstraZeneca, the manufacturer of Diprivan, states in its product labeling that the drug is intended for general anesthesia or monitored anesthesia care sedation and that the drug should be administered only by persons trained in the administration of general anesthesia and not involved in the surgical/diagnostic procedure. (For sedation of intubated, mechanically ventilated adult patients in the ICU, product labeling notes that the drug should be administered only by persons skilled in managing critically ill patients and trained in cardiovascular resuscitation and airway management.)

Unpredictable and Profound Effects:
Propofol dosing and titration are variables based on the patient's tolerance to the drug. Profound changes can occur rapidly. A patient can go from breathing normally to a full respiratory arrest in seconds, even at low doses, without warning from typical assessment parameters.[2]

No Reversal Agent:
There is no reversal agent for propofol, unlike other sedation agents such as midazolam and fentanyl; therefore, adverse effects must be treated until the drug is metabolized.

Financial Incentives:
The unwillingness of insurers to reimburse anesthesia care for some procedures such as diagnostic endoscopy has increased the use of nurse-administered propofol (1,2). Untrained nurses may be caught in the middle of the debate and feel pressured to administer Propofol.[2]

Legal Barriers:
Nurse-administered propofol falls under each state's Nurse Practice Act (i.e., Scope of Practice). More than a dozen states specifically consider this function beyond the scope of nursing practice. [2]

Safe Practice Recommendation:
At each organization, an interdisciplinary team, including chair of the anesthesia department, should establish policies and practice guidelines for administering propofol (or other induction agents such as thiopental, methohexital, etomidate, or ketamine) to nonventilated patients undergoing surgical or diagnostic procedures. To best inform your team's decision about this controversial issue, consider the following:

Review regulations/position statements: Check with your State Board of Nursing to determine if nurse-administered propofol is deemed within the professional nurses' scope of practice. If so, explore the various position statements available on this topic from professional societies, including the:

- American Society of Anesthesiologists (ASA).
- American Association of Nurse Anesthetists (AANA).
- American Association of Moderate Sedation Nurses (AAMSN).
- American Association for Accreditation of Ambulatory Surgery Facilities (AAAASF).
- American College of Gastroenterology (ACG).
- American Gastroenterological Association (AGA).
- American Society for Gastrointestinal Endoscopy (ASGE).
- Society of Gastroenterology Nurses and Associates (SGNA).

- In brief, the ASA, AANA, and AAAASF believe that only persons trained in the administration of general anesthesia, who are not simultaneously involved in the procedures, should administer Propofol to nonventilated patients. The ASA also suggests that, if this is not possible, non-anesthesia staff who administer propofol should be qualified to rescue patients whose level of sedation becomes deeper than intended and who enter, if briefly, a state of general anesthesia. The ACG, AGA, ASGE, and SGNA endorse nurse-administered propofol under the direction of a physician if state regulations allow it, and if the nurse is trained in the use of drugs causing deep sedation and capable of rescuing patients from general anesthesia or severe respiratory depression.

- **Define policies**: Based on patient safety, professional association position statements, and applicable state laws, determine the qualifications of professionals who can administer Propofol to nonventilated patients during procedures. If nurse administered Propofol is acceptable, specify the circumstances and required education and mentorship that must be accomplished beforehand, and competencies that must be evaluated and met periodically (ACLS certification alone is not sufficient (2)). Decide if the location of Propofol administration plays a factor. Location need not be limited if criteria are met, including expertise in intubating patients, which is difficult to meet in physician office settings. Define the intended level of sedation. However, even if moderate sedation is intended, all patients given Propofol should receive care consistent with deep sedation.

  Establish a continuous monitoring process and assessment criteria (e.g., vital signs, oxygen saturation, ideally capnography) for nonventilated patients who are receiving propofol. Ensure that equipment is readily accessible at the point of care to maintain a patent airway, provide oxygen, intubate, ventilate, and offer circulatory resuscitation.

Conclusion:

The debate about who should be allowed to administer propofol may continue, but one thing is clear: whenever propofol is used for sedation/anesthesia, it should be administered only by persons who are:

    (1) Trained in the administration of drugs that cause deep sedation and general anesthesia,
    (2) Able to intubate the patient if necessary, and
    (3) Not involved simultaneously in the procedure itself.

Ketamine (Ketalar)

Ketamine hydrochloride (Ketalar) – Medication used primarily for deep sedation in pediatric patients. Not a primary use drug. Administer ketamine only with previous experience or under the direction of a provider familiar with its use. Package insert "Ketamine should be used by or under the direction of physicians experienced in administering general anesthesia and in the maintenance of an airway and the control of respiration."

Mechanism of Action – Selectively interrupts cerebral pathways, causing dissociative anesthesia.

Route	Onset of Action	Peak Effect	Duration
IV	Less than 60 seconds	5 - 10 minutes	5 - 15 minutes
IM	3 - 8 minutes	5 - 20 minutes	12 - 25 minutes

Kost, p. 107, 2020

1. Dosage and Administration - usually 0.25 to 1.0 mg/kg. The dose is based on patient response to medication. The rate of infusion should not exceed 50 mcg/kg/min.

2. Adverse Reactions
   - Respiratory effects – bradypnea, dyspnea, respiratory depression, apnea, bronchial smooth muscle relaxation, increased tracheo-bronchial tree secretions.

- Cardiovascular effects – bradycardia, tachycardia, hypertension, hypotension, arrhythmias.
- Musculoskeletal – enhanced skeletal tone.
- CNS - uncontrolled muscle movements, visual illusions.
- GI – vomiting, increased salivary secretions.
- Special considerations – monitor the patient for emergent reactions, including vivid dreams or hallucinations. Consider premedication (Midazolam) to reduce the potential for adverse responses.

Methohexitol (Brevital®)
Classification: Ultra short-acting IV barbiturate anesthetic.

Anesthesia by IV: 50 – 120 mg to start; 20 -40 mg every 4 to 7 minutes (doses must be titrated to effect).
Initial dose: 0.25 – 0.5 mg / kg titrate to effect.
Duration: Single-dose 5 - 10 minutes.
Supplied: 500 mg, 2.5 g., 5 g. (powder for reconstitution).

Route	Onset of Action	Peak Effect	Duration
IV	30 seconds	45 seconds	5-10 minutes

Kost, p. 114, 2020

Etomidate (Amidate)
Classification: Sedative Hypnotic ultra-short-acting non barbiturate.

Sedation initial dose: 0.1 mg/kg IV bolus.
Additional dose: 1 – 4 mg titrate to effect.
Supplied: 2 mg/ml (10ml, 20ml) injection.

Etomidate

Route	Onset of Action	Peak Effect	Duration
IV	30-60 seconds	1-2 minutes	3-5 minutes

6. Other Sedating Medications

Diphenhydramine Hydrochloride (Benadryl)

Diphenhydramine hydrochloride is an antihistamine H1-receptor drug with anticholinergic and sedative properties. It is usually given as a premedication before endoscopic procedures to achieve a synergistic effect in combination with a narcotic and benzodiazepine, which allows for lower doses of these drugs.

Route	Onset of Action	Peak Effect	Duration
IV	2-3 minutes	60-90 minutes	240 minutes

Administer intravenously at a rate generally not exceeding 25 mg/minute or inject deep intramuscularly, not to exceed 400 mg/day. Additional doses up to 100 mg may be used as needed.

Alpha-2 Receptors Agonists

Clonidine (Catapres)

Preoperatively, Clonidine (Catapres) an alpha-2 adrenergic receptor agonist, causes sedation and reduces autonomic nervous system reflex responses. These responses may include those secondary to catecholamine release in general and hypertension and tachycardia.
Clonidine is FDA approved for Critical Care Sedation.
Dose 3-5 mcg/kg

Route	Onset of Action	Peak Effect	Duration
Oral	30-45 minutes	2-4 hours	8 hours

Omoigui, p. 34

Dexmedetomidine (Precedex)

When Precedex is infused for more than 6 hours, patients should be informed to report nervousness, agitation, and headaches that may occur for up to 48 hours. Additionally, patients should be informed to report symptoms that may occur within 48 hours after the administration of dexmedetomidine such as: weakness, confusion, excessive sweating, abdominal pain, salt cravings, diarrhea, constipation, dizziness or light-headedness.

Route	Loading Dose	Onset of Action	Maintenance Dose	Duration of Action
IV	1 mcg/kg Over 10 min	10-15 min	0.2-1 mcg/hr titrated	Half-life 2- hrs

Nitrous Oxide Mixture

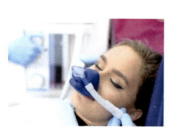 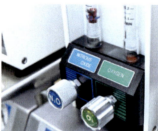

Nitrous oxide gas is used in medical and dental professions to ensure patient comfort during procedures. A 30% O_2-70% N_2O mixture is most used for sedation. The gaseous mixture, when used for sedation, is usually administered using a mask system. The onset of action for N_2O is between 2-5 minutes.

In dentistry, nitrous oxide is typically used as an anxiolytic or as an anxiety-reducing agent. N_2O is given as a 25%-50% N_2O mixture with oxygen and is most often administered through a nasal mask or nasal cannula.

The patient should be started out breathing 100% oxygen and then slowly allowed to breathe increasing amounts of N_2O until the desired effect is achieved.

Remind patients to breathe through their noses. After the procedure is finished, allow the patient to breathe 100% oxygen again for 2-5 minutes in order to clear the nitrous from the lungs.

7. Emergency Medications

Atropine / Glycopyrrolate: Increases heart rate by blocking vagal nerve stimulation. IV bolus 0.4-1.0 mg.

Produces tachycardia. Atropine or Glycopyrrolate is given to a patient with a very slow heart rate with a resultant low blood pressure.

Atropine dose:
Adult – 0.4mg – 1mg intravenous
Pediatrics – >5kg (11 lbs.) 0.01 – 0.2 mg/kg, minimum dose of 0.1mg

Route	Onset of Action	Peak Effect	Duration
IV	45-60 seconds	2 minutes	1-2 Hours
IM	5 – 40 minutes		1-2 Hours

Kost, p. 110

Glycopyrrolate does:
Adult – 0.1mg intravenous repeated every 2-3 minutes as needed.
Pediatrics – Use Atropine

Route	Onset of Action	Peak Effect	Duration
IV	45-60 seconds	2 minutes	1-2 hours

Malamed, p. 343

Lidocaine: Drug of choice for ventricular dysrhythmias - decreases automaticity. IV bolus 50-100 mg.

Route	Onset of Action	Peak Effect	Duration
IV	45-90 seconds	1 - 2 min.	10 - 20 minutes

Ephedrine: Increases blood pressure and heart rate by indirect cardiac stimulation. Slow IV push 5 - 25 mg (Adult), may repeat in 5 - 10 minutes; Pediatric dose 0.2 - 0.3 mg/kg/dose.

Route	Onset of Action	Peak Effect	Duration
IV	30 - 45 seconds	2 - 5 min.	10 - 60 min.
IM	≤ 5 minutes	< 10 min.	10 – 60 min.

Kost, pp. 110-111

Succinylcholine: IV bolus for tracheal intubation is 0.6 mg/kg. Peak effect 1 minute and persists 2 minutes.

Route	Onset of Action	Peak Effect	Duration
IV	30-60 seconds	60 seconds	4-6 minutes

The average dose required to produce neuromuscular blockade and to facilitate tracheal intubation is 0.6 mg/kg Anectine (succinylcholine chloride) injection given intravenously.

The optimum dose will vary among individuals and may be from 0.3 to 1.1 mg/kg. Following administration of doses in this range, neuromuscular blockade develops in about 1 minute; maximum blockade may persist for about 2 minutes, after which recovery takes place within 4 to 6 minutes. However, very large doses may result in more prolonged blockade.

Chapter Four

Airway Assessment

The pre-sedation assessment is both a physician and nursing responsibility and includes establishing NPO status, chief complaint, current medications, drug allergies, ancillary studies, airway evaluation, history of substance abuse or sleep apnea, medical/surgical history, concurrent medical problems, ASA status, communication ability, and physical exam. Each of these is self-explanatory, and there should be no question as to their importance.

As an illustration of the importance of the above elements in a pre-sedation assessment, there may be other missed opportunities besides procedure-related efficacy. A case involving a patient complaining of difficulty swallowing and epigastric discomfort was scheduled for an Esophagogastroduodenoscopy (EGD). The sedation nurse was a RN. The primary complaint of difficulty swallowing was ignored by the physician, admitting nurse and the sedation nurse. Secondarily, the patient also stated he was very sensitive to midazolam and had prolonged deep sedation in the past. He requested they start with one-fourth of the normal dose. When injected with the sedation analgesia medications, he asked, "What did you just give me?" The nurse stated that she had given him 2 mg of midazolam and 50 µg of fentanyl. Despite his informing the nurse about his sensitivity, the patient was given their standard medication dosage. As a result, he experienced over 48 hours of amnesia. The diagnosis after endoscopy was negative for epigastric problems, and no reason was given for his difficulty swallowing. Unfortunately, several months later, it was discovered that he had a cancerous tumor on the base of his tongue the size of a ping pong ball. The physician did not see the tumor during the EGD.

That patient was lucky, and the staff that did the endoscopy were also very fortunate that he did not have any respiratory difficulty. But the excessive dose of midazolam in conjunction with the large tongue tumor could have been disastrous.

Lesson: A simple airway exam can distinguish between safe sedation and a procedural nightmare.

Upper airway anatomy is the most common site for airway obstruction:
- Mouth
- Nose
- Pharynx
- Larynx

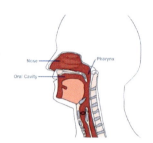

Whenever a patient is about to receive sedation, the preoperative assessment of the airway is one of the most important steps in ensuring patient safety and positive outcomes. This article, Part III in the series on airway management, is directed at the ambulatory office practice and focuses on predicting the success of advanced airway rescue techniques.

The purpose for the assessment is to determine if the patient may possibly have a difficult airway and to indicate the potential ease or difficulty of positive pressure ventilation. If assessed as having a difficult airway, it is CRITICAL that the patient maintain (protective) airway reflexes.

https://www.ncbi.nlm.nih.gov/pmc/articles/PMC4462705/

A reminder: Moderate Sedation/Analgesia

Moderate sedation is a drug-induced depression of consciousness during which patients respond purposefully to verbal commands, either alone or accompanied by light tactile stimulation. No interventions are required to maintain a patent airway, spontaneous ventilation is adequate, and cardiovascular function is usually maintained.

The following are characteristics of moderate sedation:
- Purposeful response to verbal or tactile stimulation
- No airway intervention required
- Spontaneous ventilation adequate
- Cardiovascular function usually maintained

Note:
Reflex withdrawal from a painful stimulus is NOT considered a purposeful response. Practitioners involved with moderate sedation must be prepared to "rescue" from deep sedation.

Managing the airway is the most crucial and controversial issue in non-anesthesia nurse sedation. An adequate evaluation of the airway is crucial. It is non-invasive and can be quickly completed with simple observation. The LEMON mnemonic contains the following observations for patient assessment:

L-E-M-O-N

- **L**=Look externally (facial trauma, large incisors, beard or moustache, and large tongue)
- **E**=Evaluate the 3-3-2 rule (incisor distance <3 fingerbreadths, hyoid/mental distance <3 fingerbreadths, thyroid-to-mouth distance <2 fingerbreadths)
- **M**=Mallampati (Mallampati score ≥3)
- **O**=Obstruction (presence of any condition that could cause an obstructed airway)
- **N**=Neck mobility (limited neck mobility).

Look Externally:

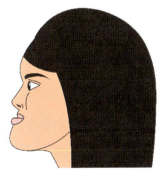
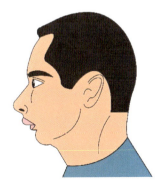

Evaluate:

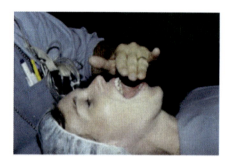
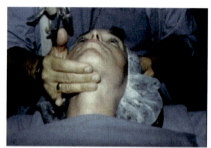

Mallampati Classification:

The Mallampati classification is a well-established assessment tool and is easy to perform and entails no cost. It is considered an accurate predictor of subtle anatomic causes that could cause difficult intubation. To perform the assessment, the patient should sit upright with the head in neutral position. The patient is then asked to open the mouth as wide as possible and to protrude the tongue as far as possible.

Classification can then be made as follows per visualization of the anatomy listed below.

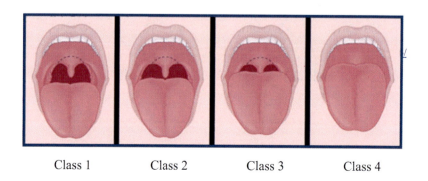

Class 1   Class 2   Class 3   Class 4

Obstruction Possibility:

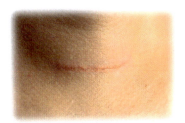
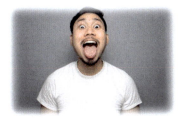

Neck Mobility:

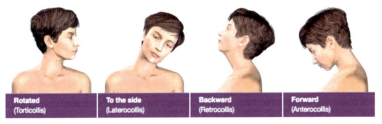

Pacific Neuroscience Institute^{SM}

Algorithm for sedation airway assessment and intervention

1. Ask patient to speak – Assessment
2. Ask patient to take a breath - Assessment
3. Head tilt chin lift - Procedure
4. Nasal Airway - Procedure
5. Oral Airway - Procedure
6. Bag valve mask positive pressure - Procedure

Chapter Five

Airway Equipment

Rescue Capacity: As stated earlier, because the level of sedation of a patient receiving anesthesia services is a continuum, it is not always possible to predict how an individual patient will respond. Further, no clear boundary exists between some of these services. Hence, hospitals must ensure that procedures are in place to rescue patients whose level of sedation becomes deeper than initially intended, for example, patients who inadvertently enter a state of Deep Sedation/Analgesia when Moderate Sedation was intended.

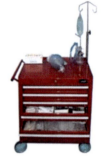

Age-specific resuscitation equipment is required to meet the emergency needs of the patient. If the facility treats pediatric patients, pediatric-sized resuscitation equipment is immediately available.

Required Equipment: The Surgical Services maintains an adequate inventory of instrumentation, supplies, and equipment. The following equipment must be available to the operating room suites:
- Call-in-system (intercom or equivalent)
- Cardiac monitor
- Defibrillator
- Aspirator (suction equipment/vacuum)
- Resuscitator (ventilator)
- Tracheotomy set
    30.00.12 Healthcare Facilities Accreditation Program (HFAP)

Additional Required Equipment for moderate sedation/analgesia
- Emergency medications
- Noninvasive blood pressure unit
- Pulse oximeter
- Capnography
- Crash cart

Oxygen must be readily available for administration by mask or nasal cannula but need not be utilized if oxygen saturation remains at a satisfactory level in the judgment of the attending provider. Monitor respiratory rate and adequacy in order to maintain oxygen saturation at a minimal SaO_2 of 95% on room air or supplemental oxygen. SaO_2 should be monitored every 5 minutes due to the potent effects of benzodiazepines and narcotics on the circulatory and respiratory systems.

Oxygen Delivery:

Nasal Cannula:
- Volume delivered via this mode is 1-6L/minute, or 24-44% concentration of O_2.
- FiO_2 is increased by 4% for each liter per minute increase in O_2 flow rate.
- Maximum FiO_2 is 44% at 6 liters/minute.
- Mouth breathing does not ablate effectiveness due to entrainment of O_2 from the nose via inspiratory air flow through the posterior pharynx.

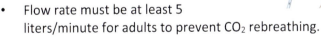

Simple Face Mask:
- Face mask is recommended for a flow of 8-10L/minute, or 40-60% concentration of O_2.
- Flow rate must be at least 5 liters/minute for adults to prevent CO_2 rebreathing.
- Maximum FiO_2 is 60% at 8 liters/minute.

Face Mask with Reservoir:
- Face mask with O_2 reservoir or non-rebreather mask is a high-flow delivery device.
- A flow of 6L/min will allow for O_2 concentrations of 60%.
- A flow of 10L/minute will allow for close to 100%.

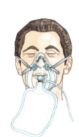

Bag Valve Mask:

- Bag-valve device is the recommended high-delivery system for acute and emergent situations. However, without experience it can be as harmful as helpful.
- Things to consider in the airway assessment that can indicate a difficult bag valve mask ventilation may include but are not limited to the following.

1. Age older than 55 years
2. Body mass index >26kg/m^2
3. Beard
4. Lack of teeth
5. History of snoring
6. Obesity
7. Mask fit
8. Proper positioning using head tilt/chin lift

For further review of airway assessment visit:
https://www.ncbi.nlm.nih.gov/pmc/articles/PMC4462705/

Airway Adjuncts:

There are two types of airway adjuncts-- the oropharyngeal airway, and the nasopharyngeal airway.

Airway adjuncts are used to relieve or bypass an upper airway obstruction during airway management. However, upper airway obstruction may be present for several reasons, and airway adjuncts may not be able to relieve or bypass all types of obstruction. Upper airway obstruction may occur from anatomical causes such as choanal atresia, pathological causes such as a tonsillar abscess or adverse effects from patient management such as loss of airway patency during the administration of sedation and/or analgesia.

Avoid using an oropharyngeal airway on a conscious patient with an intact gag reflex. If the patient can cough, they still have a gag reflex, an oral airway is contraindicated. If the patient has a foreign body obstructing the airway, an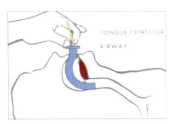
oropharyngeal airway should not be used. An oropharyngeal airway keeps the posterior pharynx open, and bypasses the tongue preventing airway obstruction by the tongue.

The correct procedure for measuring and inserting the oral airway.

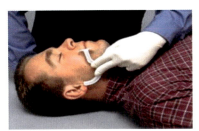 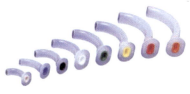

Have the patient, during the airway assessment, hold one nostril shut while breathing through the other. Choose the most patent nostril if nasal airway adjunct is indicated. Avoid using a nasopharyngeal airway on a patient with a fractured or bleeding nose.

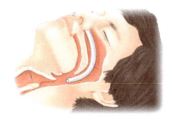

General Anesthesia:

According to Joint Commission Standard PC.12.20 EP 4 - which states that "Individuals administering moderate or deep sedation are qualified and have the appropriate credentials to manage patients at whatever level of sedation or anesthesia is achieved..."

Losing the airway is a high risk when the sedated patient enters deep sedation or general anesthesia. If the patient, becomes apneic the airway may be maintained by using a bag valve mask. However, knowing how to assemble and efficiently use the bag valve mask can be very difficult depending on your experience and what conducting the LEMON airway assessment reveals. Using the bag valve mask is a learned skill and takes practice to become proficient. Practice on a manikin as often as you can. Even, better practice with a colleague to see how well you can get a mask seal on their face.

If you fail to ventilate the patient with the bag valve mask, the next step is to intubate or place an LMA, which are learned skills. Ask yourself how prepared you are to rescue a patient in respiratory depression. You can watch a lot of videos and intubate a lot of manikins, but they do not die if the endo tube is not placed correctly through the vocal cord and into the bronchus. Moderate sedation is called moderate sedation for a reason. Moderate sedation is the average between light and deep sedation, where the patient maintains airway protective reflexes.

Chapter Six

Monitoring Vital Signs

Patient monitoring is the standard of care and indicates the patient's physiologic status. According to eh Joint Commission, the person doing the monitoring should be free of all other duties except monitoring the patient. However, the American Society of Gastrointestinal Endoscopy (ASGE) states that when the patient is receiving minimal and moderate sedation, the RN can perform short, interruptible tasks in addition to monitoring the patient.

The best monitor comes in two parts – the patient who communicates through verbal or physical response and the monitor (RN) who, through vigilance, is aware of the patient's level of sedation and their vital sign responses.

The electrocardiograph (ECG), pulse oximetry, capnography, and blood pressure monitoring are the standard of care, but are not a substitute for vigilance by the person monitoring the patient. Many adverse outcomes can be prevented by the provider supplementing the use of monitors with vigilance.

Monitoring parameters include ECG, blood pressure), respiratory rate and function, oxygen saturation, level of consciousness, skin conditions and a continuously placed IV.

The ECG allows rapid detection and treatment of dysrhythmias in those at increased risk. The ECG is also an indicator of epinephrine administration, reflection of sedation levels and anxiety. Joint Commission standards also state the ECG can be optional depending on patient medical history and type of procedure.

Monitoring the blood pressure is a good indicator of medications directly depressing cardiac function, adequacy of circulation, and hydration. The cuff size is important for accurate measurement - too large creates artificially low readings, too small creates artificially high readings. The blood pressure is measured and recorded every five minutes.

Monitoring Airway

Ventilation

Ventilation starts in the upper airway, mouth, nose, pharynx, and larynx with the movement of air between the environment and the lungs via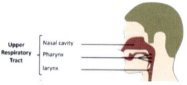
inhalation and exhalation and is the earliest indication of inadequate air exchange. The upper airway is the most common site of airway obstruction. Observation of spontaneous respiratory activity with continuous auscultation of breath sounds and having the patient talk is a good indicator of ventilation. However, oxygenation and ventilation are not synonymous. Shallow respirations with adequate oxygenation can lead to respiratory failure.

Respiration

Respiration is defined as the transport of oxygen from the outside air to the cells within tissues, and the transport of carbon dioxide from the cells in the opposite direction.

Anatomy and gas exchange does not occur in the tracheobronchial tree which is made up of the trachea and bronchi. The tracheobronchial tree is the upper conducting zone of the airway to transport air from the mouth to the alveoli. It is not where gas exchange occurs.

Anatomy and gas exchange in the lower respiratory zone consists of alveolar ducts and alveoli, the site of gas exchange. The tidal volumes must be large enough for air to reach the alveoli; otherwise, gas exchange will not occur.

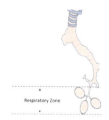

Pulse Oximetry

Pulse oximetry is the standard of care, and the perception by many healthcare providers is that pulse oximetry tells you everything you need to know. However, pulse oximetry is not a good measure of ventilation. Pulse oximetry measures oxygenation but provides you no information about ventilation. Changes in pulse oximetry can lag behind breathing changes with a delay in the onset of apnea and decreased oximeter reading - maintain VIGILANCE. A patient on supplemental O_2 with high blood concentrations of O_2 is one reason for a delay in respiration changes. Other reasons for inaccuracy may be low oxygen saturation, low perfusion states, motion, and direct ambient light.

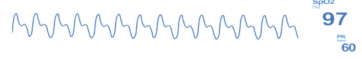

Normal Pulse OX Wave Form

Shutterstock

Capnography

- Capnometer provides a numerical measurement of carbon dioxide
- Capnogram is the waveform of carbon dioxide over a period of time.
- Capnography is the continuous measurement of the concentration of inhaled and exhaled carbon dioxide (CO2)

Capnography is proven to be a more sensitive measure of ventilation than pulse oximetry or clinical observation and is measured directly at the airway, and a presence of CO_2 equals an open airway which in return means an increase in patient safety.

Capnography provides immediate, real-time data assessment. As the respiratory rate and the depth decrease, less CO_2 is removed from the blood, which is typical during moderate procedural sedation.

Multiple organizations recommend the use of capnography in moderate sedation. The Association for Radiologic and Imaging Nurses, Association of Perioperative Registered Nurses, American Association of Moderate Sedation Nurses, and American Society of Anesthesiologists support the use of capnography.

ASA Standards require anesthesiologists to monitor $ETCO_2$ for all moderate sedations. The ASA believes that other, less-qualified, non-anesthesiologist sedation practitioners need it even more than their members to enhance their margin of safety.

Capnography respirator cycle waveform:

There are four phases of the respiratory cycle:
- Inspiratory baseline (A-B)
- Expiratory upstroke (B-C)
- Expiratory plateau (C-D)
- Inspiratory downstroke (D-E)

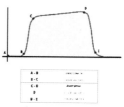

Shutterstock

End-title CO_2 ($ETCO_2$) is the concentration of CO_2 in exhaled air at the end of the expiration ($ETCO_2$ "D" circled in the graph.) Normal $ETCO_2$ is 35-45 mmHg.

What are the numeric values of capnography?

- CO_2 Less than 35 mm Hg = Hyperventilation/Hypocapnia" Ph Increases (Alkalosis)
- $ETCO_2$ Greater Than 45 mmHg = "Hypoventilation / Hypercapnia" PH Decreases (Acidosis)
- A number less than 35 means the patient is ventilated too fast and becoming alkalotic.
- A number higher than 45 means the patient is ventilated too slowly and is becoming acidotic.

Capnography provides early indications of:

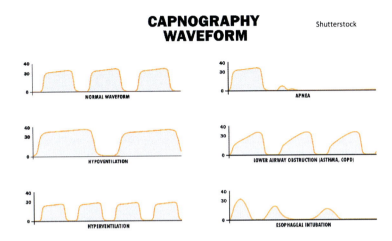

Interventions for inadequate ventilation:

- Verbally/physically stimulate the patient

- Notify the ordering provider of the patient's status

- Consider holding additional sedative medications or administration of reversal agents

- Provide head tilt/chin lift

- Reposition the head

- Consider airway adjuncts, like nasopharyngeal airway

- Call for additional help and be prepared to provide bag/mask ventilation if apnea persists

Chapter Seven

Potential Complications and Interventions During Sedation

1. **Nausea and Vomiting**

   Nausea is a subjective occurrence, and vomiting is a complex reflex involving the skeletal muscles and autonomic nervous system. The brain's chemoreceptor trigger zone (CTZ) can stimulate the vomiting center via three primary afferent nerve pathways. The three pathways are the corticoid, visceral, and vestibular afferent pathways. The causative reflexes may originate in the pharynx, GI tract, cerebral centers, or vestibular center, which controls the sense of balance. Circulating drugs or decreased cerebral blood flow can directly affect the CTZ and the vomiting center, resulting in "central vomiting." Culprit drugs include many inhalation and intravenous anesthetic agents and narcotics. With etiologic diversity, no single approach to preventing or treating nausea and vomiting will be effective from one person to another.

   Factors contributing to nausea and vomiting should be assessed and eliminated whenever possible. Interventions that may diminish potential nausea and vomiting include:

   - Provide positive reinforcement to reduce anxiety.
   - Avoid sights, smells, and conversations.
   - Move the patient slowly.
   - Allow the patient to awaken slowly without aggressive stimulation.
   - Provide adequate analgesia.
   - Provide IV access and adequate hydration.

   If vomiting occurs and the patient is obtunded or unable to protect their airway, place the patient on their side and make sure the airway is clear of vomitus. Suction as necessary. Putting the operative table in Trendelenburg position will allow gravity to drain the emesis away from the obtunded patient's trachea. If the patient is responsive and can protect their airway, they can be placed in a sitting position and given a basin.

Antiemetic therapy can reduce GI symptoms but may increase sedation. Keep in mind that Compazine (Prochlorperazine), and Phenergan (Promethazine), are classified as sedatives. Zofran (Ondansetron hydrochloride) is the least sedating of the antiemetic drug choices. Information on standard antiemetics is listed below:

Prochlorperazine (Compazine)
- Dose 5 – 10 mg IV or deep IM.
- Administration Technique: Always begin with the lowest recommended dose.
- 5 mg/minute IV. Maximum dose of 10 mg IV.
- Potential adverse reactions: drowsiness, dizziness.

Promethazine (Phenergan)
- Dose: 12.5 – 25 mg IV or 25-50 mg IM.
- Onset: 20 minutes
- Peak Action: 4-6 hours
- Duration: up to 12 hours
- Potential adverse reactions: drowsiness, dry mouth

Ondansetron Hydrochloride (Zofran)
- Dose: 4 mg IV over 2-5 minutes
- Onset: 20 minutes
- Peak Action: 3.5 hours
- Duration: up to 8 hours
- Typically, minimal side effects, but with potential for adverse reactions

2. **Respiratory Depression**
   Respiratory depression can occur because of airway obstruction or simply due to the central effects of a medication.

   Capnography and Pulse Oximetry are mechanical means for identifying early signs of respiratory depression, obstruction, and apnea. Capnography monitors ventilation, while pulse oximetry monitors oxygenation. Therefore, capnography provides breath-to-breath feedback, and changes in breathing, like apnea, are reflected immediately. Pulse oximetry measures the concentration of oxygen in the hemoglobin. However, be aware that O_2 saturation changes can lag behind breathing changes due to the effects of supplemental oxygen.

Immediate ventilatory support should be instituted for patients with shallow or absent breaths. Intervention may be administering oxygen and encouragement to breathe deeply until the effects of the sedation subsided. Elevating the patient's head and shoulders slightly may help encourage chest movement, particularly for the patient who is obese or has pre-existing respiratory compromise.

Proper positioning of the patient and suctioning the upper airway are the primary deterrents to obstruction. Until the patient can maintain an airway, constant attention must be given to the patient's head and neck position.

Airway obstruction may be partial or complete. Partial obstruction includes any degree of the following signs:
- Decreased tidal volume.
- Sternal retractions.
- Increased respiratory effort, use of accessory neck and intercostal muscles
- Abdominal breathing movements
- Decreased oxygen saturation and cyanosis (hypoxemia & hypercapnia)
- Inspiratory stridor, snoring, or gasping breath sounds

Complete respiratory obstruction results in silent, exaggerated attempts at inspiration. If not corrected, cyanosis progresses to respiratory and cardiac arrest and death.

Upper airway obstruction – A simple chin-lift/jaw-thrust can solve the problem—other interventions: auditory and tactile stimulation, head tilt, and nasal or oral airway.

In addition to proper positioning, a nasal airway may effectively correct the problem. A nasal airway tends to be better tolerated by the partially awake patient, and oxygen therapy should be administered until respiratory inadequacy has been corrected.

Auscultation is an essential part of the assessment for a sedated patient, both during the initial assessment and after attempting to arouse or reposition them. When lung sounds are difficult to hear, another helpful assessment parameter is auscultation over the trachea to check for clear and easy airflow.

3. Laryngospasm

Laryngospasm is a form of airway obstruction that can be a transient, self-limiting problem or may progress to a total obstruction that results in respiratory arrest. Intervention is usually successful in reversing the condition if detected and managed in its early stages.

Predisposing Factors:
- Stimulation of the vocal cords due to mechanical irritation by an endotracheal tube, suction catheter, or secretions may cause partial or complete laryngospasm.
- Blood or mucus from the upper respiratory tract may be a causative agent, or a foreign object may be implicated.

Symptoms:
- Dyspnea and inspiratory crowing.
- Diminished breath sounds with minimal evidence of airflow at nose or mouth.
- Awake patients who experience laryngospasm are usually terrified.
- Observation of the patient's chest is an unreliable assessment in this situation because the patient may be making vigorous yet ineffective attempts at ventilating. Vigorous attempts to breathe in the face of closed vocal cords can cause significant sternal retractions. Patients have created enough

negative intrapulmonary pressure to cause "negative pressure pulmonary edema."

Treatment:
- Immediately initiate mechanical airway maintenance and oxygen administration.
- Maintain a calm demeanor, especially if the patient is awake.
- A soothing voice, airway maintenance, and humidified oxygen may effectively break the spasm.
- If respiratory distress continues to progress, oxygen under positive pressure by bag and mask and gentle suctioning of the pharynx are indicated. Positive pressure should be applied in a prolonged, gentle, continuous manner to break laryngospasm rather than trying to ventilate the patient by repeatedly squeezing and releasing the bag. Intubation may be required if respiratory deterioration continues.

4. Bronchospasm

Bronchospasm is a narrowing of the lower airways due to increased tone in the circular smooth muscle in the bronchi or bronchioles. A bronchospasm *is a reversible event!*

Predisposing Factors:
- Asthma.
- Cigarette smoking.
- Emphysema.
- Respiratory tract infection.
- Cardiac failure.
- Allergic reaction.

Prevention:
- Obtain an accurate history and identify those at risk.
- Pre-treatment with bronchodilating agents.
- Avoid interventions that cause irritation to the tracheobronchial tree.
- Decrease anxiety and stress as a prophylactic measure.

Symptoms:
- High pitched wheezing and coarse crackles.
- Flaring nostrils.
- Increased respiratory rate and restlessness.

Treatment:
- Positioning and calm environment.
- Have the patient cough deeply with oxygen administration.
- Both inhaled and parenteral bronchodilating drugs can be used

5. **Emergence Reaction/Delirium/CNS Changes**

   Occurs during the period of arousal from general anesthesia (especially when ketamine is used). It manifests itself with behaviors such as restlessness, thrashing of extremities, combativeness, crying, moaning, screaming, irrational talking, and disorientation.

   Predisposing Factors:
   - Barbiturates and scopolamine given preoperatively are implicated as triggers.
   - Presence of pain.
   - A full bladder.
   - Feelings of suffocation and possibly cerebral hypoxia.

Prevention:
- Comprehensive preoperative preparation to establish a rapport between the patient and caregivers
- This helps reduce anxiety, encourage trust, and reduce fears surrounding surgery.

CNS Changes:
- Over-sedation or untoward reactions to the procedure or medication may occur at any time, so the patient's quality of respirations, pulse, heart rate and rhythm, blood pressure, and oxygen saturation must be assessed and documented continuously. Should untoward reactions or complications occur, initiate the appropriate supportive measures.
- Agitation and combativeness may be undesirable effects of IV sedation and can also result from hypoxemia.

6. **Drug Reactions**

   Always note allergies, be safe when administering any drugs, and titrate to effect. Maintain IV access during sedation and have Benadryl and epinephrine available at the bedside.

7. **Hypotension**

   Hypotension may result from a fluid deficit from a prolonged NPO period, inadequate intravenous replacement, medications, or blood loss. Some intravenous agents cause cardiovascular depression and decrease peripheral vascular resistance, allowing blood to pool in the extremities with a resulting drop in the mean arterial blood pressure. Investigate possible causes.

   During sedation, the blood pressure may fluctuate by 10% from baseline. A drop of 20% to 30% below the patient's normal pressure that is sustained for more than a few minutes should raise a red flag.

Treatment depends on the cause, but a combination of some or all of the following interventions may help:
- Continued oxygen therapy.
- A gentle movement of the patient.
- Supine positioning with the elevation of the legs.
- Infusion of intravenous fluids.
- Pharmacological interventions may include a vasopressor such as ephedrine or anticholinergic drugs such as Atropine.

8. Hypertension

Pain or stress of the procedure can cause hypertension, and additional sedation or analgesia may resolve this problem. Other causes include, "arousal," full bladder, hypoxemia, hypercarbia, volume overload, medications, tourniquet usage, and pre-existing hypertension.

9. Cardiac dysrhythmias

Before we get into the two common types of dysrhythmias, let's review the normal sinus heart rhythm shown in the picture.

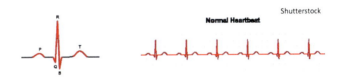

Shutterstock

The heart rate is normal (60-99 bpm), and the rhythm is regular. The QRS complex is narrow P waves are present and upright. There is a fixed 1-to-1 relationship between the P waves and QRS complexes.

The two most common cardiac arrhythmias during sedation are *bradycardia* and *tachycardia*.

More serious arrhythmias include premature ventricular contractions or atrial arrhythmias and may be caused by any of the reasons listed above under hypertension. If the patient develops new shortness of breath or chest pain, consider obtaining a 12-lead ECG immediately to determine if cardiac ischemia is present.

10. **Bradycardia**

    Sinus bradycardia is a heart rate < 60 bpm, with a P wave for every QRS.

    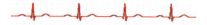

    Predisposing Factors:
    - Athletic persons.
    - Patients on Beta-Blocker therapy.
    - If not one of the above reasons, the rhythm is abnormal due to hypothermia, hypothyroidism, or sedative agents (narcotics).
    - Vagal nerve stimulation
    - Hypoxemia

    Symptoms:
    - Faintness.
    - Dizziness.
    - Decreased HR may allow for PVC's.
    - Hypotension.

11. **Tachycardia**

    Sinus tachycardia is a heart rate >100 bpm, with a P wave for every QRS.

    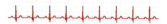

    Tachycardia can be caused by:
    - Pain
    - Anxiety
    - Hypovolemia
    - Hypoxia

12. **Cardiopulmonary arrest**

    Emergency equipment must be immediately available to the procedure room: defibrillator, code cart to include other airway devices such as laryngoscope and blades, standard resuscitation medications, age-appropriate supplies, and reversal medications (Caution: most references recommend that you have your reversal medications readily available in the procedure room itself), and back up personnel who are experts in airway management, CPR and ACLS (Anesthesia).

13. Inadequate Pain Management

Provide general comfort measures, positioning, padding, and support to the body parts. Medicate if general comfort measures do not alleviate. A soothing voice or cool cloth may be the only intervention needed to alleviate discomfort. Communication is key when interacting with the sedated patient.

Documentation Requirements During the Recovery Phase

Documentation includes the following:

Vital Signs
- Every 5 minutes during the procedure.
- Every 5 minutes times three (15 minutes), then every 15 minutes until discharge criteria are met.

Airway
- Position patient for airway observation and maintenance of clear airway.
- If the patient's face must be under drapes, be sure there is a flow of fresh air to prevent the buildup of CO_2.

Breathing
- Assess and document the rate, depth, and character of respirations.
- Monitor and document oxygen saturation. SpO2 should remain at a constant of 95% or greater regardless of oxygen delivery status.
- Record administered oxygen flow and its delivery device (face mask or nasal prongs)

Supplemental oxygen can be delivered utilizing four devices:
1. The nasal cannula is a low-flow system. The volume delivered via this mode is 1-6L/minute, or 24-44% concentration of O2.
2. A face mask is recommended for a flow of 8-10L/minute, or 40-60% concentration of O2.
3. Face mask with O2 reservoir or non-rebreather mask is a high-flow delivery device. A flow of 6L/min will allow for O2 concentrations of 60%. A flow of 10L/minute will allow for close to 100%.
4. The bag-valve device is the recommended high delivery system for acute and emergent situations.

Circulation
- Monitor pulse rate from oximeter and ECG. Good to get baseline pulse character by palpating pulse before procedure and PRN during the procedure.
- Monitor ECG for rate and rhythm. Print a pre-procedure strip and print a strip for any abnormal rhythms. If change is noted in ST segments, obtain a 12-lead ECG.
- Assess BP with vital signs. Alert physician for a sustained drop of 20% to 30% below patient's baseline.

Consciousness
- The level of consciousness is documented every 15 minutes during the procedure and in the recovery phase until the patient meets discharge criteria.
- Use the Aldrete Post-Anesthesia Scoring System to document patient LOC. Additional descriptive information can be charted to define patient status further:
    1. Alert, awake, oriented.
    2. Occasionally drowsy, easy to arouse.
    3. Frequently drowsy, able to arouse.
    4. Sleeping, slow to arouse.
    5. Somnolent, unable to arouse.

Chapter Eight

Preparation for Discharge

Increase level of activity and assess the following prior to discharge:
- Patient should be weaned to room air prior to increasing level of activity.
- Patient should progress through the phases of ambulation: elevate HOB, sit upright with legs dangling, standing upright and ambulate with a steady gait.
- Assess blood pressure prior to discharge and be aware that a lying blood pressure may give you a false sense of security. For patient safety you may also want to consider doing a sitting and standing blood pressure. Tilts should be negative (no change in blood pressure) prior to discharge. If patient is symptomatic (i.e. dizziness when standing), but tilt negative, assist patient back to bed and notify physician.

Discharge Criteria

Discharge Score

- Total score greater than or equal to 8.
- No category with a score of 0.
- Discharge policies may vary by facility.
- Data suggest the importance of discharge criteria being time based, e.g. patients must maintain wakefulness for > 20 minutes.
- **The patient must have a score of eight (8) without a zero (0) before the patient can be discharged.**

Modified Adult Aldrete Discharge Criteria Score

1. Alert & oriented to person, place, & time.

2. Stable vital signs and stable SaO_2 without supplemental O_2 for at least 30 minutes after last narcotic, sedation or hypnotic medication.

3. Pain is well controlled & easily managed with oral medications.

4. No protracted nausea/vomiting.

5. Written and verbal release instructions given to the patient. No IV sedation in the past 30 minutes.

6. Patient released in the company of a responsible adult.

7. Provide 24-hour emergency contact phone number.

8. Return inpatients to their room when considered stable and acceptable for routine ward monitoring.

9. Documentation of release criteria on flow sheet.

Modified Adult Aldrete Table

Vital Signs	Normal	2	Stable	1	Unstable	0
Respirations	Normal	2	Shallow	1	Apnea	0
Circulation	BP +/- 20 mm Hg	2	BP +/- 20-50 mm Hg	1	BP +/- 50 mm Hg	0
Consciousness	Alert	2	Arousable	1	Blunted verbal / physical	0
O_2 Saturation	94-100%	2	88-94%	1	Less than 88%	0
Ambulation	Stand	2	Vertigo when erect	1	Dizziness when supine	0
Activity	Normal	2	Altered	1	No movement	0
Pain	Pain free	2	Minimal	1	Requires meds	0
Dressing	Dry	2	Wet stationary	1	Wet growing	0

Chapter Nine

Pediatric Age-Specific Considerations

Pediatric Patients: It is suggested that patients through 18 years of age be considered pediatric patients. Intravenous sedation may be performed on pediatric patients greater than nine months of age who are assessed Class I or Class II using the Physical Status Classification of the American Society of Anesthesiologists (ASA) System.

1. **Cardiovascular System:**
    - IV cannulation of pediatric veins can be difficult. The saphenous vein at the ankle is consistent in location and serves as a viable option even when it cannot be seen or felt.
    - All air bubbles are removed from pediatric IVs since paradoxical air embolism may occur through a patent foramen ovale in pediatric patients.
    - Deep sedation, respiratory obstruction, or painful procedures may result in rapid respiratory and cardiovascular decompensation in the pediatric patient.

2. **Respiratory System:**
    - Neonates and infants have several anatomic differences from adult patients that make them vulnerable to airway obstruction: proportionately larger head and tongue; larynx positioned more anterior and cephalad; short neck and trachea; long, u-shaped, stiffer epiglottis; small mandible; redundant upper airway lymphoid tissue; small nares; and a prominent occiput puts head in a flexed position during airway management (corrected by slightly elevating shoulders with towels and placing head on donut shaped pillow).
    - Posterior displacement of the tongue may result in severe airway obstruction. A small amount of edema may greatly decrease the diameter of the pediatric airway.

- The presence of small alveoli through early childhood results in decreased lung compliance. The neonate has very limited oxygen reserves during apneic periods, and hypoxia develops quickly.
- Airway assessment is of paramount importance when evaluating the pediatric patient prior to sedation. Patients having any of the following factors that may be associated with difficulty in airway management should be referred to anesthesia:
  - History: Previous problem with anesthesia or sedation, stridor, snoring or sleep apnea, dysmorphic facial features (e.g. Pierre-Robin syndrome, trisomy 21), advanced rheumatoid arthritis.
  - Physical exam: Significant obesity (especially involving the neck and facial structures), short neck, limited neck extension, neck mass, cervical spine disease or trauma, tracheal deviation.
  - Mouth: Small opening (<3 cm), edentulous, protruding incisors, loose or capped teeth, high arched palate, macroglossia, tonsillar hypertrophy, nonvisible uvula.
  - Jaw: Micrognathia, retrognathia, trismus, significant malocclusion.

Age-Related Changes in Vital Signs for Children

Age	Respiratory Rate	Heart Rate	Arterial BP	
			Systolic	Diastolic
Neonates	40	140	65	40
12 months	30	120	95	65
3 years	25	100	100	70
12 years	20	80	110	60

(Source: Morgan, GE, Jr. and Mikhail, MS. (1996). *Clinical Anesthesiology*. Stamford, Connecticut: Appleton and Lange, p. 727.)

3. **Developmental Considerations**

    The nursing and medical staff administering sedation to the pediatric patient face the challenge of obtaining the trust and cooperation of the patient. An understanding of developmental stages and coping behaviors is essential in caring for pediatric patients. The following table on the next page provides basic information on developmental considerations for pediatric patients.

Developmental Mechanisms of Pediatric Patient Rapport

Age	Developmental Stage	Mechanism of Pain Control	Characteristics of Pain Response
Infant (1-12 mos.)	Trust vs. mistrust	Cuddling, suckling, parental presence	Generalized body response (tensing, stiffening); crying; facial tension; cannot anticipate impending pain
Toddler (1-3 yrs)	Autonomy vs. Shame and doubt	Parental presence; allow objects of security (blanket or toys); clearly delineate end of procedure (all done, no more, etc.)	Crying; physical resistance to stimulus
Preschool (2-5 yrs)	Initiative vs. Guilt	Teach and explain prior to procedure; positive reinforcement; parental presence; use of storytelling, books	
School age (5-12 yrs)	Industry vs. Inferiority	Teach and explain prior to procedure; positive reinforcement; parental presence	
Adolescent (13-19 yrs)	Identity vs. Role Diffusion	Explain Procedure	

(Source: Kost, M. (1998). *Manual of Sedation*. Philadelphia: W.B. Saunders, p. 158.)

4. **Pre-Operative Assessment:**
   - All pediatric patients scheduled to undergo sedation must have a health history and brief physical examination completed prior to the initiation of sedation.
   - This assessment should include; history of allergies, history of exposure and/or adverse reactions to parenteral sedative/analgesic medications or IV contrast material, medical history to include pertinent cardiac, pulmonary, hepatic and renal review of systems, and review of any preliminary lab tests. The ASA physical status is assigned to the patient at this point. In the pediatric patient population, the parent will usually provide significant health history information on the patient, especially with younger patient populations.
   - The interview time provides the opportunity to establish rapport with the child and parent and begin to initiate pre-procedure teaching.

5. **Pre-procedure Assessment:**
   - Past and Current Medical and Surgical History:
     - CNS: neurologic diseases, increased ICP, presence of VP shunt.
     - Neuromuscular diseases associated with weakness.
     - Pulmonary: asthma, reactive airway disease, recent or current URI.
     - Cardiac: congenital heart disease, patent foramen ovale.
     - GI: esophageal reflux (risk of aspiration), dentition or oral anomalies.
       - GU: pregnancy status.
       - Renal.
       - Hepatic.
     - Age and weight.
     - Allergies and previous adverse drug reactions or sensitivities.
     - Current drug use – include OTC, recreational and/or herbal drug use.

- Recent exposure to communicable diseases.
- Summary of previous hospitalizations.
- Past surgical history.
- Summary of previous anesthetics or history of sedation and any adverse reactions
- Family history.
- Any family history of adverse reaction to anesthesia or sedative drugs
- Physical exam:
    - Vital signs: TPR, BP, SpO2.
    - Weight, if not provided by history.
    - Congenital malformations, especially involving the head, neck, and oral cavity
    - Airway exam.
    - Heart and lung sounds
    - Physical development
- ASA Classification
- Name, address, and phone number of the child's or family's physician

6. **Pre-Procedure NPO Guidelines for Pediatric Patients:**

A documented history of oral intake will be obtained prior to procedural sedation. What follows are recommended guidelines:

Oral Intake Guidelines for Elective Sedation: Society for Pediatric Sedation 2010

Food	Hours of Fasting Required
Clear Liquids	2h
Breast Milk	2 or 4 depending on mother's diet
Formula or Light Meal (no fat)	6h
Full Meal with fat	8h

7. **For the Emergency Patient:**
   Evaluate food and fluid intake prior to the use of sedation. When protective airway reflexes are lost, gastric contents may be regurgitated into the airway. Therefore, patients with a history of recent oral intake or with other known risk factors, such as trauma, decreased LOC, extreme obesity, pregnancy, or bowel motility dysfunction should have the procedure delayed for the appropriate period of time or should be referred to Anesthesia. Some of these patients may benefit from meds that reduce gastric volume and acidity.

8. **Monitoring Guidelines for Pediatric Sedation:**
   - TPR, BP, O2 saturation will be monitored and documented before the administration of medication and at least every 5 minutes during procedure.
   - Oxygen must be available for administration by face mask or nasal cannula but need not be used if oxygen saturation remains >95%.
   - Patient cardiac monitoring will be continued into the recovery period and until discharge criteria are met.
   - Restraining devices should be checked to prevent airway obstruction or chest restriction. If a restraint device is used, a hand or foot should be kept exposed.
   - The child's head position should be checked frequently to ensure airway patency.
   - If IV fluids are to be administered secondary to a prolonged NPO period, hourly fluid maintenance is accomplished with a balanced salt solution (Lactated Ringers or 0.45% normal saline solution). Hourly maintenance fluid requirements are calculated utilizing the 4-2-1 rule (Morgan & Mikhail, 1996, p. 728):
     - 4 ml/kg/hour for the first 10 kg of weight.
     - 2 ml/kg/hour for the second 10 kg of weight.
     - 1 mg/kg/hour for each remaining kg of weight.

Example: 25 kg child
- 4 ml x 10 kg x 1 hour = 40 ml/hour.
- 2 ml x 10 kg x 1 hour = 20 ml/hour.
- 1 ml x 5 kg x 1 hour = 5 ml/hour.

Total = 65 ml/hour (hourly maintenance fluid rate).

Pre-procedure volume deficits are also often replaced. The example above is that a 25 kg child has a 65 ml/hour maintenance fluid requirement. If the NPO period for this child was 4 hours, then the volume deficit is 65 ml/hr X 4 hrs NPO = 260 ml.

9. **Pharmacologic Differences of the Pediatric Patient:**
Pediatric patients have different absorption, metabolic, and elimination rates that are both age-related and individual for each patient. Effects of a drug are related to each patient's developmental, physical, and chemical makeup. Some special rules apply when administering drugs to pediatric patients:
- Look each drug up in a reliable pediatric resource for dose confirmation.
- Check and have someone else recheck your dose calculations.
- **Always titrate the dose of the drug to individual patient response.**

10. **Post-Procedure Monitoring:**
- Effects of medications will last beyond the end of the procedure. Therefore, appropriate monitoring and, if necessary, emergency treatment must be utilized in the post-procedure period.
- Patients who have received antagonist agents (e.g., Naloxone or Flumazenil) must be monitored for an extended period because the reversal effect is always shorter than the effect of the drugs being reversed.
- Documentation criteria for vital signs and LOC are the same as for adults.

11. **Discharge Criteria:**
    For the young or disabled patient, the following criteria must be based upon the patient's pre-sedation level of function. Patient status at the time of discharge will be documented in the medical record:
    - Cardiovascular function and airway patency are satisfactory and stable.
    - Patient is easily arousable and protective reflexes are intact.
    - Patient can talk (if age and developmental stage appropriate).
    - Patient can sit up unaided (if age appropriate).
    - For the very young or disabled individual, the pre-sedation level of consciousness or one as close as possible to the normal level for that individual should be achieved.
    - State of hydration is adequate.
    - Scores 9-10 on the Aldrete Post-Anesthesia Score for discharge.

12. **Post Procedure Discharge Instructions:**
    - Should be provided to the responsible adult.
    - Instructions should include any limitation of activity, dietary modifications, medications, and information for follow-up.
    - A telephone/pager number should be provided to call in the event of complications.

For more information and training in pediatric sedation go to:

https://www.pedsedation.org/

Chapter Ten

Geriatric Age-Specific Considerations

Age may bring wisdom, but it also brings a greater chance of developing health problems, some of which might require surgery. Being older also affects the way your body reacts to surgery and anesthesia. Half of all people 65 and older will have at least one surgical procedure. The non-anesthesia provider is responsible for understanding the differences in how seniors may respond to medication given for anxiolysis and sedation to safely and effectively control procedure-related pain. (ASA Seniors and Anesthesia)

- Beginning of late adulthood/geriatrics is 65 years and older.
- Functional age is more important than chronological age.
- Decline in organ function is responsible for the physiologic aging process.
- Careful titration and reduced doses of medications are required to avoid the development of deep sedation states, prolonged recovery, and cardiovascular depression.

Overview

- Beginning of late adulthood/geriatrics is 65 years.
- Functional age is more important than his or her chronological age.
- Decline in organ function is responsible for the physiologic aging process.
- Careful titration and reduced doses of medications are required to avoid the development of deep sedation states, prolonged recovery, and cardiovascular depression.

Cardiovascular System Changes:

⇓ Tissue elasticity, which results in increased BP.
⇑ Systolic BP secondary to ventricular hypertrophy and decreased arterial wall compliance.
⇓ Cardiac output by 1% for each year after 30.
⇑ Cardiac dysrhythmias secondary to degenerative changes of the cardiac conduction system.
⇓ Baroreceptor activity.
Careful monitoring of urine output, fluid and electrolyte imbalances, BP, and heart rate is essential.
Caution should be taken during IV fluid infusions to avoid fluid overload with resultant CHF.

Pulmonary System Changes:

⇓ Total lung capacity
⇓ Vital capacity
⇓ PaO_2
Altered ventilation response to hypercapnia and hypoxia
⇑ Residual volume
⇑ Dead space
Laryngeal and pharyngeal reflexes are diminished.

Renal System Changes:

⇓ Glomerular filtration rate
⇓ Creatinine clearance
⇓ Tubular function (excretion)
⇓ Renal clearance of drugs and metabolites are more prone to dehydration & electrolyte imbalance.

Hepatic System Changes:

⇓ Hepatic blood flow due to decreased cardiac output
⇓ Microsomal enzyme activity
⇓ Ability to metabolize drug; prolonged effect of meds; as much as 30% from middle adult to late adult age

Gastrointestinal System Changes:

⇑ Gastric emptying time (slower passage, higher incidence of reflux)

Central Nervous System:

⇓ Peripheral, motor, sensory, and autonomic nerve fibers result in a decreased rate of signal processing within the brain stem and spinal cord.
- Impaired transport of amino acids and neuropeptides, which causes neurogenic atrophy
- Higher activation thresholds needed for special senses such as vision, hearing, touch, smell, pain, and temperature.

⇓ Cerebral blood flow.
⇓ Cerebral oxygen uptake.
⇑ Sensitivity to central nervous system depressant drugs.
⇓ Response to and recovery from stress, decreased functional reserve.

Psychological:

- Many geriatric patients are used to daily routines.
- Administration of sedation for a diagnostic procedure or minor surgical procedure removes the patient from this specific pattern of behavior.
- Lack of autonomy may lead to increased levels of frustration and feelings of confusion.
- Most geriatric patients do not respond well to fast-paced, disorganized practice settings.
- By identifying specific patient needs, a thorough pre-procedure assessment, and a timely explanation of the planned procedure, many geriatric patients experience the administration of sedation positively.

Considering the above considerations, moderate sedation can safely be administered to the elderly population. The definition of elderly is a subjective term but by chronological age is 65. That is, each patient should be considered as a person with different physiologic and psychologic needs. Special attention must be given to ensure a safe environment for induction of sedation. The patient should be fully assessed, keeping in mind the physiologic changes that accompany aging. Elderly patients have an increased variability of drug response and may have a decreased requirement for opioids and benzodiazepines between 30% to 50%. Add this to the fact that elderly patients have an increased redosing interval can lead to a drug overdose by the provider. Continuous monitoring for signs of intolerance and cautious administration of sedation will help reduce the risks associated with sedation in the elderly. Titration of medication is imperative in the sedation of seniors.

The number of people aged 65 and older in the United States on July 1, 2015, was 47.8 million people who utilize 14% of total federal government spending at the cost of $582 billion, including surgeries. https://www.pgpf.org/budget-basics/medicare

According to a 2018 U.S. Census Bureau report, in 2035, there will be 78.0 million people 65 years and older compared to 76.4 million under the age of 18. In other words, the elderly population will outnumber children for the first time in the country's history — a demographic shift that poses a unique set of public health challenges (Jun 21, 2018).

The airway of elderly patients may be more challenging due to the redundant oropharyngeal tissues, which can cause obstruction, and arthritis in the mandibular joint causing limited mouth opening. Arthritis may cause a limited range of motion in the neck as well. Poor dentition may affect the provider's ability to secure the airway and even more important is the edentulous patient who is not wearing their dentures which makes it difficult to maintain an airway during an apneic episode, usually caused by the cheeks sinking into the space usually occupied by the teeth or dentures. Usually, placing a four folded 4x4 between the cheek and gum will fill the space making the mask fit more easily.

Examples of aging-associated diseases are atherosclerosis and cardiovascular disease, cancer, arthritis, cataracts, osteoporosis, type 2 diabetes, hypertension, and Alzheimer's disease. The incidence of all these diseases increases exponentially with age.

As we explore the top health conditions of adults over the age of 65 associated with sedation and surgery or other invasive procedures which may start in a diagnostic lab with minimal or moderate sedation. Regardless of the sedation location, the standards for patient safety are the same.

The physical and mental assessment is the same as discussed in the nursing assessment in chapter two and includes heart disease, heart failure, heart attack, and heart arrhythmia can cause the heart to beat ineffectively and impair circulation. These conditions are associated with or caused by diabetes, high blood pressure, smoking, an improper diet, lack of exercise, and family history.

Michael Kost reports on the *geriatric syndrome,* which may include the following:
- Cognitive dysfunction
- Delirium
- Fatigue
- Malnutrition
- Sleep disorders
- Sensory and motor deficits
- Unstable gait

Cancer of all kinds, including breast cancer, colon cancer, and skin cancer, fall into this category. The malignant blood and bone marrow diseases that cause leukemia are also part of this group. Older adults are at greater risk than the general population for cancer though the cause is unclear.

In conclusion, administering moderate procedural sedation by a non-anesthesia nurse trained in safe and effective sedation for geriatric patients is nothing outside the RN's scope of practice and basic nursing skills. Certification in Advanced Cardiac Life Support (ACLS) takes on a different meaning when working with seniors. Starting an IV on a geriatric patient may be more difficult; therefore, training, experience, practice, and confidence will decrease stress and anxiety for the nurse and the patient. RNs should review their state board of nursing standards and the accreditation organization standards for guidance.

Chapter Eleven

The Power of Suggestion: The Language of Nursing

"The difference between the right word and the almost right word is the difference between lightning and the lightning bug."
— Mark Twain

Florence Nightingale first mentioned the language of nursing in her book *Notes on Nursing*. She stated, "words are great tools" (Nightingale, 1859).

Nursing is the most trusted of all professions. Unfortunately, as many nurses and nurse anesthetists talk to their patients, they are not aware of how the use of language impacts that trust. Language creates perceptions, and those perceptions are real to the patient. Biological research done by Bruce Lipton, Ph.D., describes how changing thinking changes the brain, which changes behavior or physiological response. His research demonstrates that words can transform pain and the healing process (Lipton, 2006). The brain responds equally to negative (toxic) suggestions and positive, reassuring (therapeutic) suggestions. Every suggestion creates a physiological or biochemical response, as we know when people blush from an embarrassment, wake up in a cold sweat from a nightmare, or as simple as thinking of eating a lemon.

When are patients most receptive to suggestions? During sedation and anesthesia, medications classified as hypnotics may be given to patients to decrease anxiety. Benzodiazepines (e.g., midazolam) and alkylphenols (e.g., propofol) are classified as hypnotics. Patients receiving hypnotic medications are more responsive to what they hear and see. Therefore, patients are more receptive to hypnotic suggestions during the procedural period when hypnotic medications are pharmacologically active. During this period, the brain responds to the suggestions, creating a biological and physiologic reaction.

A person in pain, fear, or panic is considered in an altered state of consciousness. Healing suggestions can be spoken to the body and accepted as reality by the brain, which releases proteins to maintain what was suggested, such as you are more comfortable than you thought you would be.

Words may affect the following functions:

✓ Pain	✓ Bowel motility
✓ Heart Rate	✓ Smooth muscle
✓ Contractions	✓ Sweating
✓ Blood pressure	✓ Allergic responses
✓ Bleeding	✓ Asthma
✓ Inflammation	✓ Immune response
✓ Itching	✓ Other responses

Very simply, negative or toxic language creates negative perceptions and negative emotional and/or physical responses.

Examples of Toxic Language:

- This may burn...
- You may feel an electric shock down your spine.
- It's really noisy in the operating room.
- This will feel like a little bee sting.
- That equipment is broken again?!
- How much pain are you having on a scale of 0-10?
- Do you feel sick?
- We're going to put you to sleep.
- Are you having labor pains?
- Don't worry."
- Hurt or pain
- The doctor is cutting.
- We're putting you to sleep.
- It won't belong.
- Are you having pain? Labor pains or contractions
- Are you feeling sick?

Words paint mental pictures, change behaviors, and alter symptoms or sensations. The subconscious mind does not reason; it responds to images created by the words we speak and hear.

Examples of Positive Language

- I will be with you during the entire procedure, doing everything needed to keep you safe and comfortable.
- I will give you medications during your procedure to keep you comfortable and create good feelings in your stomach.
- You should wake up feeling comfortable and pleasantly hungry.
- Think of a happy place and imagine you are there.
- You may feel some warmth in your IV as this medicine goes in. That feeling will help you relax.
- You should wake up comfortable. If not, let us know, and we will give you some comfort medication.
- It looks like you are experiencing another "baby hug."

Suggestions should be positive and affirming, clear and specific, firm, believable, rich in imagery, and beneficial. Suggestions should avoid anger or blame. In other words, don't say, "Boy, you really broke yourself up," or "How could you do something so stupid?" Also, avoid any negative words like *pain* and *hurt*.

I recently went for blood work, and the phlebotomist said, "Sit down and roll up your sleeve. I am going to be your worst enemy today." I asked why. She said, "Because I am going to hurt you." She could have said: "Relax, this won't take long. You may not even feel it."

I use the following language in the holding area for surgery, but it could be used anywhere to reframe the patient's thinking. I ask, "Is there someplace you would rather be than here?" When they say, "Yes," I ask, "Where would you rather be?" When they tell me, I simply say, "Go there and create that place in your imagination."

Anesthetic medications such as Propofol and Versed are classified as hypnotic drugs, and these medications may magnify comments made during sedation and anesthesia. So, I often use these phrases to help my patients:

Also, remember that environmental and background noises affect patient outcomes, especially in critical care areas. We often carry on our conversations, forgetting that the hospital is more than just a workplace and that patients are sensitive to noise and can eavesdrop on our conversations.

I recommend we listen without being judgmental, avoid unnecessary noise, keep areas quiet and professional, and use softer tones. Avoid jargon; keep it simple without talking down to patients or families. We as nurses can change and enhance patient outcomes simply by the language we use and how we listen.

"How very little can be done under the spirit of fear."
- Florence Nightingale

DON'T SAY	DO SAY
This isn't going to hurt.	You might feel pressure.
Don't give up.	Focus on what feeling good would feel like.
Don't be afraid.	What are your concerns?
A little bee sting. (There is no such thing as a little bee sting.)	I little pinch.
This is going to hurt.	Some people feel this, and some people don't.
Do you feel like vomiting?	You may have a warm hungry feeling in your stomach.
We're going to put you to sleep.	I am giving you some medication that may make you sleepy
Don't worry, you won't wake up!	I will be with you the entire time to make sure you stay sedated during your surgery.
Are you feeling better?	You look/sound like you are feeling better.
See if this nitroglycerin tablet will help.	Take this. It will make you feel more comfortable.
Has the oxygen helped your breathing?	I see that the oxygen is making it easier for you to breathe.
Labor pain or contraction	Experiencing Baby Hugs

The benefits of music in the sedation setting?

The benefits of music in health care have been widely reported in the literature. Using headphones with biorhythmic music increases relaxation and decreases the noise and conversations the patient may hear in the holding area and during the procedure. Adding subliminal suggestions for moderate sedation patients may also be beneficial. In 1984 the author recorded 26 subliminal phrases that were repeated every 6 minutes for the duration of the procedure. Battery operated players and headphones with the foam pads removed and placed over a patient headcover maintained cleanliness. See examples below of phrases. These phrases are heard above biorhymic music (60 beats a minute) for general anesthesia, and during I.V sedation, the music was louder than the phrases. P\hrases should be in the first person and examples following:

- I am relaxed and comfortable.
- My surgery is going well.
- I am healing more quickly than I thought I would.
- I am feeling better than I thought I would.
- My stomach is warm and comfortable.

Patients undergoing surgery who listen to soothing talk and music while under anesthesia may wake up feeling less pain and require less pain medicine.

German researchers randomly assigned 385 surgery patients to one of two groups. The first wore earphones during their operations, listening to an audiotape that played soothing background music along with positive suggestions about the safety and success of the procedure. The second group wore earphones that played a blank tape. The anesthetist put the earphones on the patients after they were asleep and removed them before they awoke. Neither the patients nor surgeons knew who got the blank tapes. The study is in BMJ.

Of those who listened to the music and talk, 70 used no opiates at all, compared with 39 in the control group. Fifty patients in the audible tape group used non-opioid pain relievers compared with 75 of the controls. And average pain scores two hours after the operation were 25 percent lower in those who heard soothing words and music compared with those who did not.

The lead author, Dr. Ernil Hansen, a professor of anesthesiology at the University of Regensburg, calculated that for every six patients using the earphones, one would need no opiates at all after an operation.

NIH Commitment
Music has gained interest for its therapeutic value and has become a subject of scientific review at the national level. Music, categorized as a Mind-Body intervention by the NIH Institute of Alternative Medicine, has been recognized as a cost-effective, quality-focused choice. The current attitude toward the use of holistic alternatives provides a positive environment for innovative research with music. This philosophy has supported NIH awards to projects such as Music and Jaw Relaxation by Marion Good (1995).

Conclusion:
Every thought we have affects some organ or gland in our body. Imagine eating a lemon, and you experience the salivation and the tart tanginess in your parotid gland. In the same way, negative thoughts (worry) can make us sick and positive thoughts can make us well. Florence Nightingale directed nurses to use words to help patients change their thoughts. Words are still the most powerful tool a nurse has.

Incorporating many of the recommendations in this sedation guide provides the sedation practitioner with various methods to improve patient care through the power of suggestion. Each strategy suggested to a patient can affect their outcome positively or negatively, and the patient can benefit from incorporating positive suggestions and therapeutic language outlined in this chapter.

"Words are, of course, the most powerful drug used by mankind."
- Rudyard Kipling

References

1. Barash, P. G. (1991). *Handbook of Clinical Anesthesia.* Philadelphia: J. B. Lippincott Company.
2. Davis, A. G. (2013). *A Nursing Guide to Adult Moderate Sedation.*
3. Eslinger, M. R. (2016-2018). *Moderate Sedation/Analgesia, Fourth Edition.* Clinton, TN: Healthy Visions.
4. Gooden, C. K. (2018). *The Pediatric Procedural Sedation Handbook.* New York, NY: Oxford University Press.
5. *Guidelines for Sedation and Anesthesia in GI Endoscopy,* Volume 87, No. 2: 2018 Gastroenterology Endoscopy
6. Joint Commission 2001 TX.2
7. Kelley, M. S. (2003). *Monitoring Level of Consciousness.* Aspect Medical Systems.
8. King, M. a. (1986 and Reprinted in1990). *Primary Anaesthesia.* New York: Oxford University Press.
9. Kost, M. (2004). *Moderate Sedation/Analgesia, Second Edition.* St. Louis, MO: Saunders An Imprint of Elsevier.
10. Kost, M. (2020). *Moderate Procedural Sedation and Analgesia.* St. Louis, Missouri: Elsevier.
11. Lang, M. E. (2009). *Patient Sedation Without Medication.* Trafford Publishing.
12. Lapham, R. (2015). *Drug Calculations for Nurses, Fourth Edition.* Boca Raton, FL: Taylor & Francis Group, LLC.
13. Malamed, S. F. (2010). *Sedation A Guide to Patient Management, Fifth Edition.* St. Louis, MO: Mosby Elsevier.
14. Mueller, R. A. (1988). *Manual of Drug Interactions for Anesthesiology.* New York, NY: Churchill Livingstone Inc.
15. Nagelhout, J. J. (1997). *Handbook of Nurse Anesthesia.* Philadelphia: W. B. Saunders Company.
16. Odom-Forren, J. a. (2005). *Practical Guide to Moderate Sedation/Analgesia, Second Edition.* St. Louis, MO: Elsevier Mosby.
17. Omoigui, S. (1991-2013). *Anesthesia Drugs Handbook, Fourth Edition.* Hawthorne, CA: Sota Omoigui.
18. Skelly, M. a. (2003). Conscious Sedation. London and Philadelphia: Whurr Publishers, Ltd.
19. Smith, D. F. (2001). *Sedation Anesthesia, and the JCAHO, Second Edition.* Marblehead, MAOmoigui's SOTA: Opus Communications, Inc.
20. Twersky, R. S. (1995). *The Ambulatory Anesthesia Handbook.* St. Louis, Missouri: Mosby-Yearbook, Inc.
21. Valente, T. (2010). *Capnography King of the ABC'S.* Bloomington, IN: iUniverse.
22. Voogd, Sarah (2019). *Capnography for Procedural Sedation: What Pulse Oximetry Cannot Tell You.* Presentation AAMSN Conference, Palm Springs, CA 2019
23. Wiener-Kronish, J. P. (2001). *Conscious Sedation.* Philadelphia, PA: HANLEY & BELFUS, INC.

Appendix

Suggested Competency Model

This competency model is a validation mechanism for registered nurses taking the Certified in Sedation Registered Nurse course. It is intended to help nurses assume the multifaceted role of the Sedation Nurse.

The competency module is a self-paced program designed to accommodate the various clinical experiences each nurse may possess with sedation. Successful achievement of this entire module is necessary to be considered competent in management of the sedated patient.

Phase I
- Review the position statement and acknowledge your role in the management of patients receiving sedation.
- Review your current institution's policy on sedation. If no policy exists, use sample policy provided in the Appendix to develop a formal policy for your institution.

Phase II
- Complete the Sedation Certification Seminar (CSRN) prior to clinical practicum.
- Concentrate on acquiring knowledge in the field of physiology and pharmacology related to sedation.

Phase III
- When possible spend time in Surgery, Outpatient Surgery, Endoscopy and/or Oral Surgery Clinic to observe and become familiar with the role of the sedation nurse during the pre-procedure assessment, intra-procedure monitoring and post-procedure recovery period.
- Accompany an anesthesia provider to the Operating Room to experience at least 2 airway management procedures and become familiar with airway techniques.

Phase IV
- Complete at least five (5) sedation procedures with preceptor (physician, nurse anesthetists, or qualified nurse) in order to obtain skills necessary to perform independent demonstration of competency.

Phase V
- Complete "post-test" with score of 80% or better
- Course evaluation.

Non-Anesthesia Providers Administering Sedation

Suggested Prerequisites

1. *Current license as RN, MD, PA, DDS or Podiatrist (see facility policy for others qualified).
2. *Current ACLS or PALS Certification.
3. *Successful completion of a sedation course with a post-test passing grade of 80% or better.
4. IV Insertion certificate or a part of job description from facility recommended.
5. IV Push certificate or listed in job description by facility recommended.
6. Institutes Medication Certification recommended.
7. Five sedation cases supervised by CSRN, CRNA or Physician recommended.
8. Completion of 2 airway management experiences with anesthesia personnel in the operating room, if available. If not available, documentation of completion of an airway hands on class, simulator or a comprehensive airway education video.

* Required

Moderate Sedation for Non-Anesthesia Nurses

Competency -Tool Part 1

The following assessment tool is a recommendation and can be adopted to meet the requirements of your facility.	
Insert Your Logo and Facility Information	Sedation Clinical Competency Assessment
Name:	Employee Number:
Department:	Department:
Job Title:	Date(s) of event:
A competency demonstration is usually a planned activity in which staff are asked to demonstrate skills for the purpose of assessment. The technique is effective in verifying both learned competencies and those that require psychomotor skills (i.e. demonstrating vital signs, hand washing or IV Start). Competency demonstrations can take place at the bedside or in a skills lab.	
Clinical competencies for sedation/analgesia is a demonstration of knowledge in the following areas and any other areas the institution determines is appropriate: - Goals, definitions, practice standards and guidelines of accrediting body, state and facility - Presedation assessment and patient selection - Sedation equipment checks, suction, O2, Ambu, etc. - Pharmacology concepts, sedation/analgesia medications, rescue medications and techniques of administration - Monitoring requirements - Airway assessment and management to include airway adjuncts - Age related considerations of the geriatric and pediatric patient - Risk management strategies	

Clinical Competency Assessment Demonstration Criteria	Performed
Description and/or steps as appropriate for the competency demonstration:	
1. Demonstrates knowledge of state legislature, state BON, institution, and accrediting bodies policy and position statement on non-anesthesia RNs and sedation	☐Yes ☐No
2. Gathers and prepares all supplies for monitoring patient	☐Yes ☐No
3. Prepares medications for moderate sedation/analgesia	☐Yes ☐No
4. Reviews orders, patient's history and physical and informed consent	☐Yes ☐No
5. Assesses NPO status	☐Yes ☐No
6. Educates patient on moderate sedation procedure	☐Yes ☐No
7. Confirms availability of emergency equipment and medications	☐Yes ☐No
8. Recognizes structures of the oral airway (Mallampati 1-4)	☐Yes ☐No
9. Is able to assess the different ASA 1-6 classifications.	☐Yes ☐No
10. Attaches monitoring equipment correctly	☐Yes ☐No

Moderate Sedation for Non-Anesthesia Nurses

Competency Tool - Part 2

The following assessment tool is a recommendation and can be adopted to meet the requirements of your facility.			
Insert Your Logo and Facility Information	Sedation Clinical Competency Assessment		
11. Establishes IV access and verbalizes that IV access is maintained throughout procedure and recovery phase		☐ Yes	☐ No
12. Demonstrates knowledge of medication dosages, administration, and adverse reactions of medication.		☐ Yes	☐ No
13. Assesses and monitors patient during moderate sedation • Verbalizes documentation frequency of vital signs documentation during moderate sedation (minimum of 5 minutes) • Respiratory rate • Oxygen saturation • Blood Pressure • Cardiac Rate • Level of consciousness		☐ Yes	☐ No
14. Verbalizes when to report VS assessment to physician and need for patient intervention • Oxygen saturation • Dyspnea • Symptomatic Bradycardia/Hypotension • Seizures • Cardiac Arrest		☐ Yes	☐ No
15. Demonstrates interventions to support patient that has an adverse event from medication administration		☐ Yes	☐ No
16. Recognizes airway obstruction and demonstrates skills in BLS i.e. Head tilt chin lift, placement of an Oral airway and/or nasal airway.		☐ Yes	☐ No
17. Demonstrates use of the positive pressure device and suction equipment		☐ Yes	☐ No
18. Verbalizes completion of the Medication Safety Form (if patient receives a reversal agent		☐ Yes	☐ No
19. Demonstrated sedation criteria for geriatric and pediatric patients		☐ Yes	☐ No
20. Verbalizes post procedure patient assessment • Vital Sign frequency (minimum of every 5-15 minutes) • Recovery time for patient receiving reversal agent • Discharge criteria score		☐ Yes	☐ No

☐ Competency demonstrated   ☐ Not yet deemed competent, action plan required (indicated below)
Action Plan:

Validator signature: _____   Date: _____

Employee signature: _____   Date: _____

Supervisor/Manager signature: _____   Date: _____

Sample of Informed Consent

1. I_____(Patient's name), acknowledge that I am scheduled to undergo a procedure and request that I be given sedation medication to relieve anxiety and pain.

2. Sedation for my procedure has been explained to me by_____, and I have had all my questions concerning sedation explained to my satisfaction.

3. I understand that in addition to the risks of the procedure, sedation carries its own risks. Complications that arise include, but are not limited to, the following:

    a. Nausea/vomiting
    b. Damage to blood vessels
    c. Respiratory problems
    d. Drug reactions
    e. Infection
    f. Heart injury
    g. Death
    h. Damage to fetus if pregnant

4. I understand that during sedation, conditions may arise which require invasive actions. I therefore authorize hospital personnel to act on my behalf.

5. I understand that my sedation will be monitored by an individual who has completed sedation training as per hospital policy and under the supervision of a credentialed physician.

6. I have received an explanation of the proposed sedation plan and have been given the opportunity to ask questions about it as well as alternatives. The risks and hazards have been explained to me, and I feel that I have sufficient information to give this informed consent.

7. I certify that this form has been fully explained to me, that I have read it, or have had it read to me, and that I understand its contents.

_____
Signature (Patient or person authorized to consent)
　　　Date/time

_____
Witness signature
　　　Date/time

_____
Signature and stamped name (sedation nurse)
　　　Date/time

Moderate Sedation for Non-Anesthesia Nurses

Sample Sedation Monitoring Record

Proposed Procedure		Age	Weight (kg)	Height (in)	Physical Status 1 2 3 4 5 E	Allergies
Chemistries	**Hematology** H / H - Platelets - WBCs -	**Coags** PT - INR - PTT -	**Urinalysis / HCG**		**Airway assessment:**	
Respiratory Tobacco: Cough: Sputum: Asthma: COPD: Recent URI: TB: CXR: Lung Exam:	**CV** HTN: CAD: MI: CHF: VHD: Arrhythmias: Exercise Tolerance: ECG: Cardiac Exam:		**CNS / Skeletal** Seizure: CVA: LOC: Neuro: Muscle: Skeletal: **Misc** BP: HR:		**Other** Hepatic: Renal: GI: Esophageal Dz.: Thyroid: Diabetes: Heme: EtOH:	

Previous Anesthetics/Complications:	Current Medications:
Family Hx: **Preoperative Diagnoses** 1. 2. 3. 4. 5.	**Day of Procedure:** ☐ Chart Reviewed / Patient examined ☐ Risks / benefits / options discussed with patient ☐ Patient questions answered ☐ Patient / parent / guardian understands and accepts risks ☐ NPO after _____ liq., _____ clears, _____ solids **Sedation nurse signature** **Date & Time** Comments:
Patient identification	Post-procedure note ☐ No apparent complications from sedation. Signature Date/Time

Conscious Sedation Pre/Post-Procedure Summary

SAMPLE SEDATION MONITORING RECORD	Allergies:	Weight:

Procedure:
Date: | Start Time: | Stop Time: | Surgeon:

Time

- ● = Pulse
- ○ = Spont Resp
- V = Sys
- ∧ = Dia

Pre-Procedure VS
Pulse
BP
HR
SaO_2

SaO_2
Verbal
Cardiac Rhythm
O_2 L/M
Meds:

Total dose _____
Total dose _____
Total dose _____

Post Procedure Record

Medications Used	Route	Total	Fluids		Discharge vital signs:
			Type	Amount	Pulse:
					Heart Rate:
					Blood Pressure:
			EBL		Pulse Ox:
			Urine		

Time	Notes:

Discharge Criteria: Normal Color, Fully Awake, Breathes freely and deeply, Able to move all unrestricted extremities, Blood pressure within 20% of pre-procedure level

Identification:

Post Procedure Documentation
- ☐ Meets all discharge criteria
- ☐ Written instructions given
- ☐ Discharged to care of responsible adult
- ☐ UNABLE TO MEET DISHARGE CRITERIA
  (Patient care turned over to PACU)

Sedation Provider Signature: _____ Date/Time: _____

Patients Receiving Sedation Recommendations

1. Arrangements must be made for a responsible adult to drive you home after your sedation.
2. No solid food 6-hours prior to procedure. Light meals only up to 6-hours after sedation.
3. May provide formula up to 6-hours and breast milk up to 4-hours before procedure.
4. May drink clear liquid (water, apple juice) up to 2-hours before procedure.
5. Patient may take medications with sips of water as recommended by their physician.
6. Any regular daily medications can be taken the day of your procedure, with a sip of water.
7. If you are taking medications that affect blood clotting, ask your doctor if you should stop taking them prior to your appointment.
8. You will be released to return home after your procedure, when the effects of the sedation have worn off (usually in 1-2 hours). Remember, a responsible adult (18-year-old or older) must accompany you home.
9. An adult should be with you for 24 hours and check on you frequently for the first 6-8 hours.
10. Certain sedative medications can cause difficulty with urination, which may (rarely) require catheterization of the bladder.
11. Occasionally, patients experience allergic reactions to sedative medications, including itching, rash, breathing difficulty, or other symptoms. Be sure you let your physician know your allergies.
12. You must not drive a motor vehicle, operate heavy equipment, or drink alcohol for at least 24 hours after your sedation.
13. You may experience some nausea and vomiting, but most people do not.
14. If you experience any problems or complications, notify your doctor at the number on your discharge information.
15. You may call or report to a hospital Emergency Department if needed.

Dilaudid®

Hydromorphone HCl
Analgesic – Antitussive

Action and Clinical Pharmacology: Hydromorphone has a strong analgesic action and antitussive activity. Small doses of hydromorphone produce effective and prompt relief of pain, usually with minimal nausea and vomiting. Generally, when given parenterally, hydromorphone's analgesic action is apparent within 15 minutes and remains in effect for more than 5 hours. The onset of action of oral hydromorphone is somewhat slower, with measurable analgesia occurring within 30 minutes. When sleep follows the administration of hydromorphone, it is due to relief of pain, not to hypnosis.

Hydromorphone is approximately eight times more potent on a milligram basis than morphine. In addition, hydromorphone is better absorbed orally than is morphine; the former is approximately 20 to 25% as active orally.

Hydromorphone has greater antitussive potency than codeine on a weight basis. However, its dependence liability is also greater than that of codeine.

After absorption hydromorphone is metabolized by the liver to the glucuronide conjugate which is then excreted in the urine.

Indications and Clinical Use: Relief of moderate to severe pain.

Contra-Indications: Intracranial lesion associated with increased intracranial pressure, status asthmaticus, and pulmonary edema.

Precautions: May be habit-forming. Hydromorphone is a narcotic with an addiction liability similar to that of morphine and for this reason the same precautions should be taken in administering the drug as with morphine.

Pregnancy: As with all narcotics, hydromorphone should be used in early pregnancy only when expected benefits outweigh risks.

If necessary, hydromorphone may be given IV, but the injection should be given very slowly. Rapid IV injection of narcotic analgesic agents, including hydromorphone, increases the possibility of adverse effects, such as hypotension and respiratory depression.

As with any narcotic analgesic agent, the usual precautions should be observed, and the possibility of respiratory depression should be kept in mind. If a patient shows signs of hypersensitivity to hydromorphone, the treatment must be stopped.

Dilaudid injection has been reported to be physically or chemically incompatible with solutions containing sodium bicarbonate and thiopental sodium.

Children: Hydromorphone suppositories are not recommended for use in children.

Adverse Reactions: Nausea, vomiting, dizziness, somnolence, anorexia, and constipation may occur. Pain at the injection site; local tissue irritation and induration following s.c. Injection, particularly when repeated in the same area.

Symptoms of Overdose: Serious overdose with hydromorphone may be characterized by respiratory depression (a decrease in respiratory rate and/or tidal volume, Cheyne-Stokes respiration, cyanosis), extreme somnolence progressing to stupor or coma, skeletal muscle flaccidity, cold and clammy skin, and sometimes bradycardia and hypotension. In severe over-dosage apnea, circulatory collapse, cardiac arrest, and death may occur.

Treatment: If significant respiratory depression occurs, it may be antagonized by Naloxone as recommended by the manufacturer. Employ other supportive measures as indicated.

Dosage: Orally for adults, 2 to 4 mg every 4 to 6 hours as required. The usual adult parenteral dose for pain relief is 2 mg by subcutaneous or intramuscular routes every 4 to 6 hours as necessary. If necessary, hydromorphone may be given IV, but the injection should be given very slowly. Severe pain can be controlled with 3 to 4 mg every 4 to 6 hours as necessary. Rectal suppositories (3 mg) provide long-lasting relief and are especially useful at night.

The oral liquid may be diluted in fruit juice or other beverage, if desired.

IV Initial: Opiate-naive: 0.2-0.6 mg every 2-3 hours as needed; patients with prior opiate exposure may tolerate higher initial doses. Dilute 2mg one ml ampoule into 9cc's of saline, which is 0.2mg per ml.

Note: More frequent dosing may be needed.

Mechanically ventilated patients: 0.7-2 mg every 1-2 hours as needed; infusion (based on 70 kg patient): 0.5-1 mg/hour.

Patient-controlled analgesia (PCA):
Opiate-naive: Consider the lower end of the dosing range.
Usual concentration: 0.2 mg/ml
Demand dose: Usual: 0.1-0.2 mg; range: 0.05-0.5 mg
Lockout interval: 5-15 minutes
4-hour limit: 4-6 mg

Epidural:
Bolus dose: 1-1.5 mg
Infusion concentration: 0.05-0.075 mg/ml
Infusion rate: 0.04-0.4 mg/hour
Demand dose: 0.15 mg
Lockout interval: 30 minutes

Note: Intramuscular use may result in variable absorption and a lag time to peak effect.

Initial:
Opiate-naive: 0.8-1 mg every 4-6 hours as needed; patients with prior opiate exposure may require higher initial doses; usual dosage range: 1-2 mg every 3-6 hours as needed.

Precedex

Precedex is indicated for sedation in non-intubated patients prior to, during surgical and other procedures, intubated, and mechanically ventilated patients during treatment in an intensive care setting.

Precedex should be administered by continuous infusion not to exceed 24 hours.

Caution should be exercised when administering Precedex to patients with advanced heart block and/or severe ventricular dysfunction.

Clinically significant episodes of bradycardia, sinus arrest and hypotension have been associated with Precedex infusion and may necessitate medical intervention.

Initiation and maintenance dosing

Precedex is generally initiated with a loading dose of 1 mcg/kg over 10 minutes for both procedural sedation and ICU sedation.

However, coadministration of Precedex with anesthetics, sedatives, hypnotics, and opioids can enhance the pharmacodynamic effects of these agents. Specific studies have confirmed these effects with sevoflurane, isoflurane, Propofol, Alfentanil, and Midazolam. Therefore, a decrease in the dosage of Precedex or the concomitant agent may be required.

In patients already sedated with other anesthetics, sedatives or opioid analgesics, a loading dose may not be necessary.

Prior to initiating a loading dose, consideration should be given to the existing level of sedation and the condition of the patient.

For ICU sedation: Maintenance dosing of Precedex is initiated at 0.4 mcg/kg/hr. and titrated over a dose range of 0.2 to 0.7 mcg/kg/hr.

For sedation during surgical and other procedures: After administration of a 1 mcg/kg loading dose, the maintenance dose of Precedex is initiated at 0.6 mcg/kg/hr. and titrated to achieve the desired clinical effect, with doses ranging from 0.2 to 1 mcg/kg/hr.

http://www.precedex.com/dosing/dosing-basics/

CSRN™ Scope of Practice

Certified Sedation Registered Nurse (CSRN)

Certification is a process by which a nongovernmental agency validates, based upon predetermined standards, an individual nurse's qualifications and knowledge for practice in a defined functional or clinical area of nursing.

Certified Sedation Registered Nurses (CSRNs™) are registered nurses who become sedation certified by taking an advanced curriculum of study that focuses on developing knowledge in the areas of patient assessment, pharmacology, airway, monitoring, equipment, emergencies, and emergence, clinical judgment, and critical thinking. It is within the scope of practice of a registered nurse to manage the care of patients receiving sedation during therapeutic, diagnostic, or surgical procedures under the guidance of a licensed independent provider (LIP) who is qualified by education, licensure, and certification.

CSRNs are legally responsible for the sedation care they provide, which is determined by their state Board of Nursing (BON) policy and position statement on non-anesthetist's RNs giving sedation. If there is no BON policy on non-anesthesia RNs giving and monitoring sedation, then guidance should come from their facility sedation policy and their job description. More information concerning state policies can be found at:

http://sedationcertification.com/resources/position-statements/position-statements-by-state/clickable-map/

Responsibilities and Functions:

The Scope of Practice of CSRNs includes, but is not limited to, the following:

1. Administration of moderate sedation medications by non-anesthetist RNs is allowed by state laws and institutional policy, procedures, and protocol.

2. A qualified anesthesia provider or attending physician selects and orders the medications to achieve moderate sedation.

3. Guidelines for patient monitoring, drug administration, and protocols for dealing with potential complications or emergency situations are available and have been developed in accordance with accepted standards of anesthesia practice.

4. The registered nurse managing the care of the patient receiving moderate sedation shall have no other responsibilities that would leave the patient unattended or compromise continuous monitoring.

5. The registered nurse managing the care of patients receiving moderate sedation is able to:

   a. Demonstrate the acquired knowledge of anatomy, physiology, pharmacology, cardiac arrhythmia recognition, and complications related to moderate sedation and medications.

   b. Assess total patient care requirements during moderate sedation and recovery. Physiologic measurements should include, but not be limited to, respiratory rate, oxygen saturation, blood pressure, cardiac rate and rhythm, and patient's level of consciousness.

   c. Understand the principles of oxygen delivery, respiratory physiology, transport, and uptake, and demonstrate the ability to use oxygen delivery devices.

   d. Anticipate and recognize potential complications of moderate sedation in relation to the type of medication being administered.

   e. Possess the requisite knowledge and skills to assess, diagnose and intervene in the event of complications or undesired outcomes and to institute nursing interventions in compliance with orders (including standing orders) or institutional protocols or guidelines.

    f. Demonstrate their `skill in airway management resuscitation.

    g. Demonstrate knowledge of the legal ramifications of administering moderate sedation and/or monitoring patients receiving moderate sedation, including the RN's responsibility and liability in the event of an untoward reaction or life-threatening complication.

6. The institution or practice setting has an educational/competency validation mechanism that includes a process for evaluating and documenting the individuals' demonstration of the knowledge, skills, and abilities related to the management of patients receiving moderate sedation. Evaluation and documentation of competence occur periodically according to institutional policy.

Additional nurse sedation responsibilities which are within the expertise of the individual CSRN™ may include the following:

1. Administration/management: scheduling, material, and supply management, development of policies and procedures, fiscal management, performance evaluations, preventative maintenance, billing, data management, and supervision of staff, students, or ancillary personnel.

2. Quality assessment: data collection, reporting mechanism, trending, compliance, committee meetings, departmental review, problem-focused studies, problem-solving, interventions, documents, and process oversight.

3. Education: clinical and didactic teaching, BCLS/ACLS instruction, in-service commitment, and facility continuing education.

4. Research: conducting and participating in departmental, hospital-wide, and university-sponsored research projects.

5. Committee appointments: assignment to committees, committee responsibilities, and coordination of committee activities.

6. Interdepartmental liaison: interface with other departments such as nursing, surgery, obstetrics, post sedation care units (PACU), outpatient surgery, admissions, administration, laboratory, pharmacy, etc.

7. Clinical/administrative oversight of other departments: respiratory therapy, PACU, operating room, surgical intensive care unit, pain clinic, etc.

The functions listed above are a summary of CSRN™ clinical practice and are not intended to be all-inclusive.

Sample Procedural Policy for Sedation

- Place your Facility Information Here -

MODERATE SEDATION

1. **Purpose.** To establish minimum requirements for administering and monitoring sedation and establishing "one standard of care" for all patients throughout this facility, utilizing guidelines established in references (a) and (b).
    a. Patients in the Special Care Unit on ventilators.
    b. Patients under age 12.
    c. Situations requiring sedation/analgesia for patients who are not undergoing a diagnostic/therapeutic procedure (i.e., pain control or treatment of insomnia).
    d. Situations where the clinician's intent is to provide anxiolysis, using standard recommended doses of benzodiazepines alone or in combination with a narcotic.
    e. Circumstances that require the assistance of a qualified anesthesia provider, including:

    (1) Situations requiring sedation during which it is anticipated that the required sedation will eradicate the purposeful response to verbal commands or tactile stimulation and/or result in partial or complete loss of protective airway reflexes including the ability to independently maintain a patent airway.

    (2) Preoperative management of patients undergoing general anesthesia or major conduction blockade.

2. **Cancellation.** See or create institution policy

3. **Definition.** Sedation is produced by the administration of drug(s) which depress the level of consciousness (with or without providing analgesia) while retaining the ability to independently and continuously maintain a patent airway

and to respond appropriately to verbal and physical stimuli. Adequate respiratory drive is maintained.

4. **Patient Evaluation.**
    a. The need for any short-term therapeutic, diagnostic, or surgical procedure and subsequent use of sedation will be directed by a credentialed physician and/or dentist.

    b. Practitioners are required to consult with an anesthesia provider when there is a question regarding the appropriate delivery of sedation.

    c. Patients (or their legal guardians) will be informed of the risks and benefits of sedation and agree to its administration. Informed Consent and Authorization for Sedation form will be used to obtain written informed consent.

    d. Patients undergoing sedation for elective procedures should adhere to the following NPO guidelines put forth by the anesthesia department: no solids for six hours prior to scheduled procedure and stop clear liquids two hours prior to scheduled procedure to allow gastric emptying.

    e. A Sedation Pre-Procedure Evaluation must be completed and included in the medical record. Post-procedure care must be documented on the Sedation Monitoring Record.

    f. Constant monitoring of the patient is required to assess the level of sedation and to ensure the safety of patients undergoing procedures requiring sedation.

5. **Practitioners.**
    a. The minimum number of available medical personnel for any procedure employing sedation will be two. The operator (physician or dentist performing the procedure(s)) and the monitor (an assistant formally trained to administer medications and sedation under the direction of the operator, to monitor appropriate physiologic parameters, and to assist in supportive or resuscitative measures as required). However, the monitor shall have no other duties. These personnel will be available to the patient from the time of administration of sedation until recovery is complete. When needed, a third person will be used to assist and or circulate during the procedure.

    b. The operator is required to hold current credentials and facility privilege as established by the facility and granted by administration.

    c. The provider performing the procedure will verify that all Practitioners who perform sedation have completed an Advanced Cardiac Life Support course.

    d. The operator selects, orders, and signs the order for the medication to produce sedation.

    e. The sedation monitor must complete a sedation course, be able to monitor and react appropriately to the patient's responses to medication and at a minimum, changes in:

           (1) Vital signs.
           (2) Level of consciousness.
           (3) Airway status.
           (4) Oxygen saturation.

    f. The monitor will not engage in any tasks that would compromise continuous patient assessment. (e.g. circulation, assistant).

6. **Equipment.**
   a. The following equipment must be present, in working order, and ready for use in the room where sedation is being administered:

      (1) Oxygen
      (2) Suction
      (3) Emergency airway equipment
      (4) Non-invasive blood pressure (BP) monitor or manual BP cuff
      (5) Pulse oximeter
      (6) Cardiac (EKG) monitor
      (7) Narcan and Romazicon or their equivalents.
      (8) Emergency medications

   b. A cardiac arrest cart with a defibrillator will be in close proximity to the sedation and recovery site as defined by Joint Commission standards.

   c. All patients receiving IV sedation must have a patent IV with continuous administration of IV fluids per physician's order. Patent "saline/heparin locks" are acceptable for patients with contraindication to IV fluids. **IV fluid for resuscitation should be readily available.** The physician will determine the need for IV access in patients receiving sedation by any other route of administration, e.g., oral sedation.

   d. Oxygen must be available; however, it is not required to be utilized if O_2 saturation remains greater than 95% at room air.

7. Monitoring.
   a. Minimum monitoring will include:

   (1) BP
   (2) Pulse and respiratory rate
   (3) Oxygen saturation (continuous monitoring with pulse oximetry)
   (4) Level of consciousness
   (5) EKG

   b. A Standardized Sedation Monitoring Record will be completed by the sedation monitor for all patients receiving sedation and will be included in their medical record. Documentation must include:

   (1) Beginning and end time of the procedure
   (2) Pre-medication, time, and effect
   (3) Type and amount of IV fluids
   (4) Name, dose, route, and time of all drugs given
   (5) Patient response to all drugs given, including adverse drug reactions or untoward/significant responses as well as their management and outcome.
   (6) Oxygen delivered: liters per minute and route.
   (7) BP, pulse and respiratory rates, oxygen saturation, and level of consciousness must be documented in the flowsheet at least every five minutes or more frequently as the patient's clinical needs dictate. EKG abnormalities must be documented, and a pre and post EKG strip is recommended.

8. **Post-Procedure.** Patients who receive sedation will continue to be monitored after the procedure until they are fully recovered. Patients will be "recovered" when specific criteria indicate a return to safe physiological and psychological levels. The minimum criteria for recovery are as follows:

a. Heart Rate (HR) and BP are within 20% of the pre-procedure baseline; the patient responds readily, maintains room air oxygen saturation of >95%, and is free from nausea and vomiting.
b. Minimal pain or free from pain
c. If the patient is experiencing difficulty meeting discharge criteria, they may be transferred to the post-anesthesia care unit (PACU) for further monitoring/recovery

9. **Discharge.**
    a. For patients returning to the ward, a verbal report including the following will be provided to the nurse receiving the patient:

        (1) Pre-procedure BP, HR, oxygen saturation, and level of consciousness.
        (2) Total drugs given (name, dosage, and time of the last dose).
        (3) Problems encountered during or post-procedure.
        (4) Total IV fluids and status of IV.

    b. For patients returning home, verbal and written discharge instructions will be provided to the patient and the responsible adult accompanying the patient. There must be documentation that the patient has received instructions and verbalize that they understand them.

    Instructions must include at least the following:

        (1) Information on the possible residual effects and side effects of the anesthetics and instruction on what to do and who to call for assistance /emergency.
        (2) Instructions on the advancement of diet as needed.
        (3) Restrictions on activity, if any.
        (4) Medications, if any.
        (5) Follow-up appointment.

10. **Risk Management** or other appropriate person or committee will monitor the number of cases performed. In addition, they will monitor adverse events via the variance report system. The following events should be reported as variances:

    a. Patients with oxygen saturation below 90% for greater than 1 minute
    b. Patients requiring airway resuscitation.
    c. Patients requiring cardiovascular support.
    d. Patients requiring transfer to PACU due to inability to meet discharge criteria within one hour of the end of the procedure.
    e. Usage of Narcan (naloxone) or Romazicon (flumazenil).
    f. Other adverse events. (e.g. unexpected somnolence, chest pain, behavioral problems, allergic reactions, transfer to critical care or another facility).

11. **Procedure Review.** This procedure policy will be reviewed every year and revised as necessary by the Sedation Program Manager with oversight by the Executive Board of the Provider Staff. All personnel involved in the care of patients through the Sedation Program will familiarize themselves with this sedation policy.

12. **Forms.** Sedation Monitoring Record and Informed Consent and Authorization for Sedation are to be used.

Administrator Name and Signature

Index

Accreditation for Health Care Organizations, 16
Administering Sedation, Non-anesthetists, 120
airway patency, 37
Aldrete Post-Anesthesia Scoring System, 94
Aldrete, modified adult scoring, 97
Alpha-2 Receptors Agonists, 65
Alprazolam (Xanax), 49
American Association of Moderate Sedation Nurses AAMSN, 11
American Association of Nurse Anesthetists AANA, 11
American Society of Anesthesiologists ASA, 11
Anesthesia and Surgical History, 34
Anesthesia Medications, 57
Antiemetic therapy, 85
arrest, 92
Atropine, 67
Auscultation, 87
Barbiturates, 89
Benadryl, 64, 90
Benzodiazepines, 42
Blood Pressure, 38
Bodily functions affected by words, 115
Bradycardia, 92
Bronchospasm, 88
Capnography, 85
Cardiac dysrhythmias, 91
Cardiac monitoring, 38
Cardiopulmonary arrest, 92
Cardiovascular System, 29
Care of Patients, 18
Catapres, 65
Certified Sedation Registered Nurse (CSRN), 132
Chart Review, 25
Chronic Obstructive Pulmonary Disease COPD, 30
Class I, 24
Class II, 24
Class III, 24
Class IV, 24
Class V, 25
Class VI, 25
Clonidine (Catapres), 65
CNS Changes, 89
Compazine, 85
Complications during sedation, 84
Continuous IV access, 37
Cyanosis, 40
Deep Sedation/Analgesia, 15
deepening levels of sedation, 39
Delirium, 89
Demerol, 52
Dentition, 28
Dexmedetomidine (Precedex), 65
Diabetes, 32
Diaphoresis, 40
Diazepam (Valium), 42
Dilaudid, 128
Diphenhydramine Hydrochloride (Benadryl), 64
Diprivan, 57
Discharge, 96
Discharge Criteria Score, 97
disinhibition, 38
Documentation, 39
Drug Reactions, 90
Emergence Reaction, 89
Emergency Medications, 67
Ephedrine, 68
Epinephrine, 90
Escort, 35
Etomidate (Amidate), 64
Fentanyl, 51
Flumazenil (Romazicon), 43
Flushing, 40
Gastrointestinal System, 33
General Anesthesia, 15
Glycopyrrolate, 67
Goals of Sedation, 21
Hepatic System, 33
Hypertension, 91
Hyperthyroidism, 33

Hypotension, 90
hypothyroidism, 33
Informed Consent, 35
Informed Consent form, sample, 123
Integumentary System, 34
Intra-operative Nursing Actions, 37
Intra-procedure events, 36
Joint Commission Policy, 16
Ketalar, 63
Ketamine (Ketalar), 63
Language for the holding area, 116
Laryngospasm, 87
Level of consciousness
   LOC, 38
Lidocaine, 67
Lorazepam (Ativan), 48
Mallampati Airway Classification, 31
Kost, M., 102
Medication administration, 39
Medications for Moderate Sedation, 41
Meperidine, 51
Methohexitol (Brevital®), 64
Midazolam (Versed), 42
Minimal Sedation (Anxiolysis), 14
Moderate Sedation/Analgesia, 14, 70
Monitoring and documentation, 37
Morgan, GE, Jr. and Mikhail, MS Clinical Anesthesiology, 101
Morphine Sulfate, 51
Musculoskeletal System, 34
Naloxone (Narcan), 55
Naloxone Hydrochloride (Narcan), 55
Nausea, 40
Nausea and Vomiting, 84
Neurologic System, 33
Nightingale, Language of Nursing, 114
Nitrous Oxide Mixture, 66
Ondansetron Hydrochloride (Zofran), 85
optimally sedated patient, 38
Over Sedation
   Toxicity, 22
Oxygen delivery, 37
Oxygen, supplemental, 94

Pain Management, inadequate, 93
Pallor, 40
Past facial/neck trauma
   TMJ, 28
Patient Interview, 26
Pediatric considerations, 99, 108
Pediatric discharge criteria, 107
Pediatric oral intake guidelines, 104
Pediatric patient rapport, developmental mechanisms, 102
Pediatric Patient, pharmacologic differences, 106
Pediatric post-procedure monitoring, 106
Pediatric Sedation, monitoring guidelines, 105
Permission to Administer, 20
Phenergan, 85
Physical Exam, 29
Physical Status Classification System, 23
Post-procedure (recovery) events, 36
Precedex, 65, 131
Pre-Operative Nursing Assessment, 25
Preparation for Discharge, 96
Pre-Procedure Teaching, 35
Procedural Policy for Sedation, sample, 136
Prochlorperazine (Compazine), 85
Promethazine (Phenergan), 85
Propofol (Diprivan), 57
Propofol Sedation: Issues and Recommendations, 58
Pulmonary System, 29
Pulse, 37
Pulse Oximetry, 85
Recommendations for Patients, 127
Recovery Phase documentation, 93
References, 118
Registered Nurse
   RN, 12
Remimazolam (Byfavo®), 46
Renal System, 34
Report these observations, 40

Requirements for Quality Sedation, 23
Respiratory Depression, 85
Reversal agent for Benzodiazepines, 50
Reversal Agent for Narcotics, 55
Review of Laboratory Data, 34
Role of the RN, 11
Role of the Sedation Nurse, 23
Romazicon, 50
scopolamine, 89
second nurse or associate, 11
Sedation Continuum of Care, 22
Sedation Monitoring Record, sample, 125

Sedation, definition, 11
Seven medication standards, 41
Sublimaze, 54
Succinylcholine, 68
Suggested Competency Model 5 Phases, 119
Summary form, Pre-/Post-Procedure, sample, 126
Tagamet, 42
Toxic language, examples, 115
Triazolam (Halcion), 49
Valium, 42
Versed, 42, 43, 46, 48
Zantac, 42
Zofran, 85

Made in the USA
Middletown, DE
14 April 2024

52993483R00082